Clinical Anatomy of the Face for Filler and Botulinum Toxin Injection

Hee-Jin Kim • Kyle K. Seo
Hong-Ki Lee • Jisoo Kim

Clinical Anatomy of the Face for Filler and Botulinum Toxin Injection

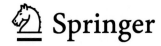 Springer

Hee-Jin Kim
Yonsei University College of Dentistry
Seoul
Republic of Korea

Hong-Ki Lee
Image Plastic Surgery Clinic
Seoul
Republic of Korea

Kyle K. Seo
Modelo Clinic
Seoul
Republic of Korea

Jisoo Kim
Dr. Youth Clinic
Seoul
Republic of Korea

Illustrations by Kwan-Hyun Youn.
Extended translation from the Korean language edition: 보툴리눔 필러 임상해부학
by Hee-Jin Kim, Kyle K. Seo , Hong-Ki Lee, Jisoo Kim
Copyright © 2015. All Rights Reserved.

ISBN 978-981-10-0238-0   ISBN 978-981-10-0240-3   (eBook)
DOI 10.1007/978-981-10-0240-3

Library of Congress Control Number: 2016938223

© Springer Science+Business Media Singapore 2016

This work is subject to copyright. All rights are reserved by the Publisher, whether the whole or part of the material is concerned, specifically the rights of translation, reprinting, reuse of illustrations, recitation, broadcasting, reproduction on microfilms or in any other physical way, and transmission or information storage and retrieval, electronic adaptation, computer software, or by similar or dissimilar methodology now known or hereafter developed.
The use of general descriptive names, registered names, trademarks, service marks, etc. in this publication does not imply, even in the absence of a specific statement, that such names are exempt from the relevant protective laws and regulations and therefore free for general use.
The publisher, the authors and the editors are safe to assume that the advice and information in this book are believed to be true and accurate at the date of publication. Neither the publisher nor the authors or the editors give a warranty, express or implied, with respect to the material contained herein or for any errors or omissions that may have been made.

Printed on acid-free paper

This Springer imprint is published by Springer Nature
The registered company is Springer Science+Business Media Singapore Pte Ltd.

Preface

First, I would like to thank my friend, Dr. Kyle Seo, for organizing all the extremely important clinical information and tips. I also wish to thank Dr. Hong-Ki Lee for his insightful inquisitions and questions that made coming up of creative contents possible. Also, I give my thanks to Dr. Jisoo Kim, who played a strong role in the planning of cadaver dissection workshops and in other works related to organizing necessary contents. Without the efforts and sacrifice of the above individuals in providing clinical manuscripts and in revising all of the visuals despite their busy clinical schedules, this book's text and artwork would not have been able to shine. As such, I send infinite thanks to Dr. Kwan-Hyun Youn for providing all of the visuals for this book. I believe that Dr. Youn, an art major graduate with a PhD in Anatomy, has raised our country's medical illustrations to that of world class. Many thanks to the effort of the Medart team led by Dr. Youn to make this book to have many clear, simple, and creative visual contents to be possible.

In the Fall of 2011, my research on clinical anatomy research in relation to aesthetics—and through this, teachings on clinical anatomy—started after receiving advice from John Rogers, a US neurology specialist and medical director of the Pacific Asian region for Allergan Inc., who visited my anatomy lab. Rogers, who had no particular interest in aesthetic treatments, enabled me to devote myself more to this field. Through regional and international educations, I had presented basic information on new methods regarding aesthetic treatment guidelines based on anatomy in order to avoid complications. Then, after hearing that many regional doctors were following anatomic guidelines based on Western research, the coauthors and I designed this book to introduce new methods to fit for Asians, who have slightly different anatomic features. For instance, Asians possess different locations of the modiolus, different directions and changes of facial arteries, and different attachment regions for muscles unlike to Caucasians. All of these and more are explained in detail in this book using research papers presented during my lectures as foundational information. Through this, new injection techniques are described in the book.

Current medical techniques are rapidly changing due to the development of science. As a result, this trend is giving way to a new slogan for medicine such as "borderless" and "above and beyond the border" for a movement working to dismantle academic borders. Biocompatible fillers and botulinum toxin injection development have started to create a new medical field of non-invasive aesthetic plastic surgery, referred to as 'Beauty Plastic Surgery', and the desire for new medical techniques is bringing about developments in clinical anatomy. Likewise, I feel that it is right for clinical doctors from all fields to come together as a virtuous group to jump over the wall of traditional medicine for the development of medical practices. And, as a health personnel studying basic medicine, I feel immense responsibility and a sense of worth in being a part of this movement.

This book includes various images and pictures for simpler understanding of anatomy from 'Plastic and Reconstructive Surgery' and other 80 research papers from acknowledged journals in relation to clinical anatomy. In addition, we worked to include various documents about Koreans so that it may be utilized as a useful document in other areas. It is my wish that, through this book, readers are able to learn clinical techniques related to aesthetic treatments and to grow in knowledge regarding the prevention of complications.

I also thank Professor Kyungseok Hu and my graduate student Sang-Hee Lee, You-Jin Choi, Hyung-Jin Lee, Jung-Hee Bae, Liyao Cong, and Kyuho Lee from Yonsei University College of Dentistry who actively helped search for visual information and aided in other revision works for this book. Lastly, I would like to thank Dr. Yoonjung Hwang, Mr. Sanghoon Kwon, Juyong Lee, Yongwoong Lee and Ms. Hwieun Hur, and Young-Gyung Kim in translating the Korean manuscript of this textbook.

On the behalf of the authors,

Seoul, South Korea   Hee-Jin Kim
November, 2015

Contents

1 **General Anatomy of the Face and Neck**.   1
  1.1 Aesthetic Terminology   2
      1.1.1 Basic Aesthetic Terminology   2
  1.2 Layers of the Face.   5
      1.2.1 Layers of the Skin.   5
      1.2.2 Thickness of the Skin   6
  1.3 Muscles of Facial Expressions and Their Actions   7
      1.3.1 Forehead Region.   8
      1.3.2 Temporal Region (or Temple).   10
      1.3.3 Orbital Region.   11
      1.3.4 Nose Region   13
      1.3.5 Perioral Muscles   14
      1.3.6 Platysma Muscle.   20
  1.4 SMAS Layer and Ligaments of the Face   21
  1.5 Nerves of the Face and Their Distributions   23
      1.5.1 Distribution of the Sensory Nerve   24
      1.5.2 Distribution of the Motor Nerve   24
      1.5.3 Upper Face   24
      1.5.4 Midface.   25
      1.5.5 Lower Face   26
  1.6 Nerve Block   28
      1.6.1 Supraorbital Nerve Block (SON Block)   28
      1.6.2 Supratrochlear Nerve Block (STN Block)   28
      1.6.3 Infraorbital Nerve Block (ION Block)   28
      1.6.4 Zygomaticotemporal Nerve Block (ZTN Block) . . .   29
      1.6.5 Mental Nerve Block (MN Block).   29
      1.6.6 Buccal Nerve Block (BN Block)   29
      1.6.7 Inferior Alveolar Nerve Block (IAN Block).   31
      1.6.8 Auriculotemporal Nerve Block (ATN Block).   31
      1.6.9 Great Auricular Nerve Block (GAN Block).   31
  1.7 Facial Vessels and Their Distribution Patterns   32
      1.7.1 Facial Branches of the Ophthalmic Artery   34
      1.7.2 Facial Branches of the Maxillary Artery.   35
      1.7.3 Facial Artery   35
      1.7.4 Frontal Branch of the Superficial Temporal Artery .   37
      1.7.5 Facial Veins.   38
      1.7.6 Connections of the Vein   42

1.8   Facial and Skull Surface Landmarks   42
1.9   Characteristics of Asian (Korean) Skull and Face   45
1.10   Anatomy of the Aging Process   48
        1.10.1 Aging Process of the Facial Tissue   49
        1.10.2 The Complex Changes of the Facial
                 Appearance with Aging   50
Suggested Reading.   51
        Physical Anthropological Traits in Asians   51
        Muscles of the Face and Neck   52
        Vessels of the Face and Neck   52
        Peripheral Nerves of the Face and Neck.   53

2   Clinical Anatomy for Botulinum Toxin Injection   55
    2.1   Introduction.   56
            2.1.1   Effective Versus Ineffective Indications
                     of Botulinum Toxin for Wrinkle Treatment   56
            2.1.2   Botulinum Rebalancing   56
    2.2   Botulinum Wrinkle Treatment   58
            2.2.1   Crow's Feet (Lateral Canthal Rhytides)   58
            2.2.2   Infraorbital Wrinkles.   62
            2.2.3   Horizontal Forehead Lines   63
            2.2.4   Glabellar Frown Lines   63
            2.2.5   Bunny Lines   69
            2.2.6   Plunged Tip of the Nose   70
            2.2.7   Gummy Smile, Excessive Gingival Display   71
            2.2.8   Nasolabial Fold   71
            2.2.9   Asymmetric Smile, Facial Palsy   72
            2.2.10 Alar Band   75
            2.2.11 Purse String Lip   75
            2.2.12 Drooping of the Mouth Corner   75
            2.2.13 Cobblestone Chin   80
            2.2.14 Platysmal Band   81
    2.3   Botulinum Facial Contouring   84
            2.3.1   Masseter Hypertrophy.   84
            2.3.2   Temporalis Hypertrophy   88
            2.3.3   Hypertrophy of the Salivary Gland   89
    Suggested Reading.   91
            Muscles of the Face and Neck   91
            Peripheral Nerves of the Face and Neck.   92
            Others   92

3   Clinical Anatomy of the Upper Face for Filler Injection   93
    3.1   Forehead and Glabella   94
            3.1.1   Clinical Anatomy   94
            3.1.2   Injection Points and Methods   94
            3.1.3   Side Effects   100
    3.2   Sunken Eye and Pretarsal Roll   103
            3.2.1   Clinical Anatomy   103
            3.2.2   Injection Points and Methods   105
            3.2.3   Side Effects   109

3.3   Temple.   109
      3.3.1   Clinical Anatomy   111
      3.3.2   Injection Points and Methods   113
      3.3.3   Side Effects.   116
Suggested Reading.   118
    Muscles of the Face and Neck   118
    Vessels of the Face and Neck   118
    Peripheral Nerves of the Face and Neck.   118

4   Clinical Anatomy of the Midface for Filler Injection   119
4.1   Tear Trough.   120
      4.1.1   Clinical Anatomy   120
      4.1.2   Injection Points and Methods   123
4.2   Nasojugal Groove   124
      4.2.1   Clinical Anatomy   124
      4.2.2   Injection Points and Methods   127
4.3   Palpebromalar Groove   128
      4.3.1   Clinical Anatomy   128
      4.3.2   Injection Points and Methods   128
4.4   Nasolabial Fold.   128
      4.4.1   Clinical Anatomy   128
      4.4.2   Injection Points and Methods   131
4.5   Hollow Cheek   135
      4.5.1   Clinical Anatomy   135
      4.5.2   Insertion Points and Methods   135
4.6   Subzygoma Depression.   138
      4.6.1   Clinical Anatomy   138
      4.6.2   Injection Points and Methods   139
4.7   Nose   139
      4.7.1   Clinical Anatomy   139
      4.7.2   Injection Points and Methods   148
Suggested Reading.   150
    Physical Anthropological Traits in Asians   150
    Muscles of the Face and Neck   150
    Vessels of the Face and Neck   151
    Peripheral Nerves of the Face and Neck.   151

5   Clinical Anatomy of the Lower Face for Filler Injection   153
5.1   Lip.   154
      5.1.1   Clinical Anatomy   154
      5.1.2   Injection Points and Methods   154
      5.1.3   Side Effects.   157
5.2   Chin.   160
      5.2.1   Clinical Anatomy   160
      5.2.2   Injection Points and Methods   160
      5.2.3   Side Effects.   162
5.3   Perioral Wrinkles   165
      5.3.1   Clinical Anatomy   165
      5.3.2   Injection Points and Methods   166
      5.3.3   Side Effects.   166

5.4   Marionette Line and Jowl 166
      5.4.1   Clinical Anatomy 166
      5.4.2   Injection and Methods. 168
      5.4.3   Side Effects............................... 168
5.5   Anatomical Considerations of the Symptoms
      That May Accompany Filler Treatment 169
      5.5.1   Vascular Compromise....................... 169
      5.5.2   Suggested Methods to Reduce Vascular
              Problems Related with Filler Injection 172
Suggested Reading..................................... 173
      Physical Anthropological Traits in Asians 173
      Muscles of the Face and Neck 173
      Vessels of the Face and Neck 173
      Peripheral Nerves of the Face and Neck................ 174

Index 175

General Anatomy of the Face and Neck

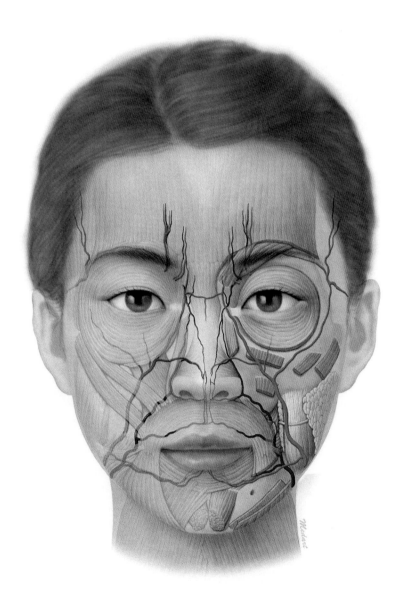

Hee-Jin Kim (Illustrated
by Kwan-Hyun Youn)

© Springer Science+Business Media Singapore 2016
H.-J. Kim et al., *Clinical Anatomy of the Face for Filler and Botulinum Toxin Injection*,
DOI 10.1007/978-981-10-0240-3_1

1.1   Aesthetic Terminology

Inconsistencies exist between anatomical and aesthetic terminology. We attempt to redefine common clinical terms according to anatomical regions (Fig. 1.1).

1.1.1   Basic Aesthetic Terminology

Facial Creases
Facial creases are deep, shallow creases caused by changes in the structural integrity of the skin. It occurs due to loss of skin and muscle fiber elasticity caused by repetitive facial movements and changes in facial expressions. Creases are generally termed wrinkles and lines. Other terms such as furrow, groove, and sulcus are used in the clinical fields.

Skin Folds
Skin folds occur due to sagging, loss of tension, and gravity. Representative skin folds are the nasolabial fold, the labiomandibular fold, etc.

Baggy Lower Eyelids (or Cheek Bags, Malar Bags)
Baggy lower eyelids occur due to a drooping of the adipose tissue underneath the orbicularis oculi m. This should be distinguished from the festoon since the baggy lower eyelid occurs inferior to the orbital margin.

Blepharochalasis
Blepharochalasis occurs due to sagging of the eyelid skin.

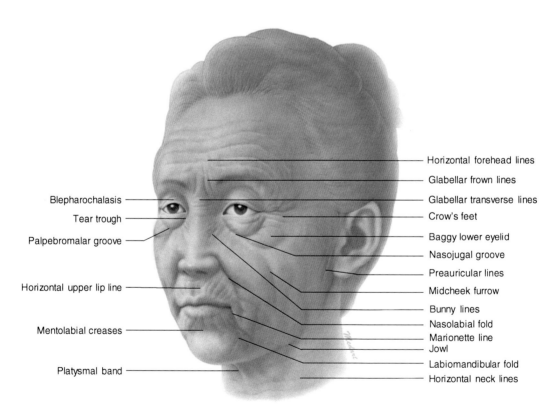

Fig. 1.1 Aging facial creases and wrinkles (Published with kind permission of © Kwan-Hyun Youn 2016. All rights reserved)

Bunny Line
The bunny line is the oblique nose furrows lateral to the nose bridge that is pronounced by various facial expressions. The levator labii superioris alaeque nasi m. below the skin and the medial muscular band of the orbicularis oculi m. participate in the formation of the bunny line.

Commissural Lines
Commissural lines are short, vertical lines appearing on each sides of the mouth corner. Occasionally, deep creases may form starting from the perioral regions.

Crow's Feet (Lateral Canthal Wrinkles)
Crow's feet are thin, bilateral wrinkles at the lateral sides of the eyes formed by the orbicularis oculi m.

Festoon
Festoon is the bulged appearance of the lower eyelids caused by a sagging of the skin and of the orbicularis oculi m. and by a protrusion of the inferior orbital fat compartment underneath the orbital septum.

Horizontal Forehead Lines (Worry Lines)
Horizontal forehead lines are horizontal lines across the forehead region where the frontalis m. is located.

Glabellar Frown Lines (Glabellar Creases or Lines)
Glabellar frown lines are vertical creases along the glabellar region caused by the corrugator supercilii muscle fibers.

Glabellar Transverse Lines
Glabellar transverse lines are horizontal lines on the radix that are typically produced during facial distortion. They occur perpendicular to the fibers of the procerus m.

Gobbler Neck (Platysmal Bands)
The gobbler neck appears as bilateral vertical skin bands on the neck along the anterior cervical and submental region. This occurs due to sagging of the medial border of the platysma muscle.

Horizontal Neck Lines
Horizontal neck lines are horizontal skin folds on the anterior cervical region. They are produced by a combination of platysmal muscle fibers and sagging neck skin.

Horizontal Upper Lip Lines (Transverse Upper Lip Lines)
Horizontal upper lip lines are 1–2 horizontal lines located at the philtrum on the upper lip.

Jowl (Jowl Sagging)
Jowl is the protrusion and sagging of the subcutaneous adipose tissue along the mandibular border. The anterior border of the prejowl sulcus clearly signifies the existence of mandibular retaining ligaments.

Oral Commissure
The labial commissure is the region where the upper and lower lips join on each lateral side. The joining point is referred to as the cheilion.

Labiomandibular Fold
The labiomandibular fold spans from the corner of the mouth to the mandibular border and becomes prominent with age. The depressor anguli oris m. (DAO) defines the fold's medial and lateral borders. The attachment of the mandibular retaining ligament causes the labiomandibular fold to be located more anteriorly and medially.

Marionette Line
The marionette line is a long, vertical line that proceeds inferiorly from the corner of the mouth.

It occurs commonly with age but with unknown causes. It is more pronounced in people with less fat tissues than in those with more fat tissues. This line is also called the "disappointment line."

Mentolabial Creases (or Furrows)

Mentolabial creases are horizontal creases (one or more) between the lower lip and the chin (mentum). These creases lie between the orbicularis oris m. and the mentalis m.

Midcheek Furrow (Indian Band)

The midcheek furrow is a downward and lateral band, or furrow, that extends the nasojugal groove from the lateral aspect of the nose to the region superior to the anterior cheek. This band may carry on inferior to the cheek. With age, the cheek and the midface droop inferiorly and medially, and the band forms along the inferior margin of the zygomatic bone at the same height where the zygomatic cutaneous ligament attaches to the skin in this region.

Nasojugal Groove

The nasojugal groove is formed at the border between the lower lid and the cheek and runs inferolaterally from the medial canthus. The nasojugal groove region corresponds with the lower border of the orbicularis oculi m. and becomes more pronounced with the existence of the medial muscular band of the orbicularis oculi m. With age, this groove obliquely continues downward to the midcheek furrow.

Nasolabial Fold (or Nasolabial Groove)

The nasolabial fold starts from the side of the nasal ala and extends obliquely between the upper lip and the cheek. With age, the subcutaneous adipose tissue of the anterior cheek sags, causing the fold to deepen and move downward. The adipose tissue of the anterior cheek cannot descend inferior to the nasolabial fold due to compact attachment of the fascia, the skin, the cutaneous insertions of upper lip elevator muscles, and the zygomaticus major m. into the skin in this area. In addition, the facial area tends to lie underneath the nasolabial fold with variable depths.

Palpebromalar Groove

The palpebromalar groove is the border between the lower lid and the malar region.

Preauricular Lines

Periauricular lines are several vertical skin lines located near the tragion, the ear lobule, and the anterior region of the auricles.

Ptotic Chin

The ptotic chin is a flat and contracted chin associated with a deepened submental crease.

Tear Trough

The tear trough is a line originating from the medial canthus and proceeding inferolaterally along with the infraorbital margin. With age, the inferior and medial portions of the orbit sink due to contraction of the soft tissues (skin, muscle, and fat) covering the area. The tear trough has various forms according to how the medial part of the orbicularis retaining ligament and the fibers of the medial muscular band of orbicularis oculi m. come into contact with the skin.

Temple Depression

Temporal depression is the gradual decrease in volume of the soft tissues of the temporal region expressed with age. The bone structure of the temporal crest becomes more pronounced.

Vertical Lip Line

As aging is processed, the tooth is lost and alveolar bone is absorbed. It leads perioral muscle and lip contracts, so the vertical lip line appears along the vermilion border.

1.2   Layers of the Face

1.2.1   Layers of the Skin

Basic facial soft tissues are composed with five layers: (1) skin, (2) subcutaneous layer, (3) superficial musculoaponeurotic system (SMAS), (4) retaining ligaments and spaces, and (5) periosteum and deep fascia. Facial skin can move over the loose areolar connective tissue layer with the exception of the auricles and the nasal ala, which are supported by the cartilage under the skin. Facial skin contains numerous sweat and sebaceous glands (Fig. 1.2a, b).

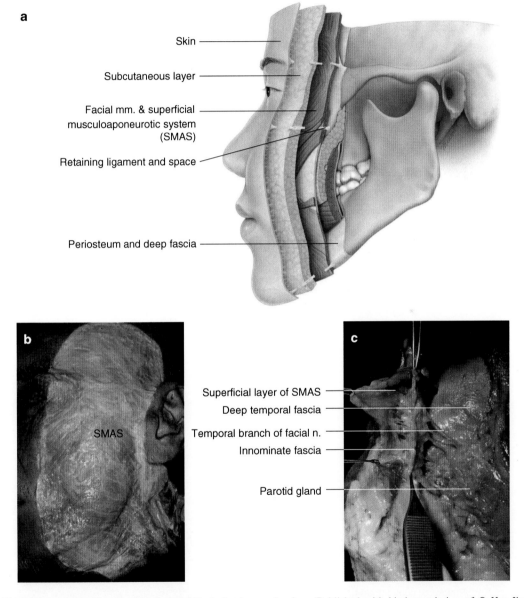

Fig. 1.2 Anatomical layers of the face. (**a**) Basic five layers of the face, (**b**) SMAS (superficial musculoaponeurotic system), (**c**) reflected SMAS at the lateral aspect of the face (Published with kind permission of © Hee-Jin Kim, Kwan-Hyun Youn and Joo-Heon Lee 2016. All rights reserved)

Among the subcutaneous fat tissue of the face, superficial fat is divided into malar, nasolabial fat, and so on. However, the boundary is not visible to the naked eye and the superficial fat may seem to cover the whole face. Deep fat is placed in the deeper part of the facial muscle and is demarcated by dense connective tissues such as the capsules or retaining ligaments. The color and properties of the deep fat show different characteristics from the superficial fat. Suborbicularis oculi fat (SOOF), retro-orbicularis oculi fat (ROOF), buccal fat, and deep cheek fat are included in the deep fat of the face. Fibrous connective tissues pass through facial fat tissues and play in role in connecting the fat tissue, facial muscles, dermis, and bone (Figs. 1.3 and 1.4).

The superficial fascia, or subcutaneous connective tissue, contains an unequal amount of fat tissue, and these fat tissues smoothen the facial contour between facial musculatures. In some areas, fat tissues are broadly distributed. The buccal fat pad forms the bulged cheek and continues to the scalp and the temple region. The facial v., the trigeminal nerve, the facial nerve, and the superficial facial muscle are contained within the subcutaneous tissue (Fig. 4.27).

The SMAS (superficial muscular aponeurotic system) is the superficial facial structure composed of muscle fibers and superficial facial fascia. It is a continuous fibromuscular layer investing and interlinking the facial m. The SMAS extends from the platysma to the galea aponeurotica and is continuous with the temporoparietal fascia (TPF, superficial temporal fascia) and the galea layer. It is known that the SMAS consists of three distinct layers: a fascial layer superficial to the muscles, a layer intimately associated with the facial m., and a deep layer extensively attached to the periosteum of facial bones (Fig. 1.2c).

1.2.2 Thickness of the Skin

The general thickness of the facial skin is described in the figure below. When treating in areas with thin layers of skin, a filler injection should be cautiously performed while trying to avoid shallow filler placement. Upper and lower eyelids, glabellar regions, and nasal regions have an exceptionally thin skin layer. On the other hand, the skin layer of the anterior cheek and the mental region are relatively thicker. During filler treatment, the skin's flexibility and internal space should also be considered along with its thickness (Fig. 1.5).

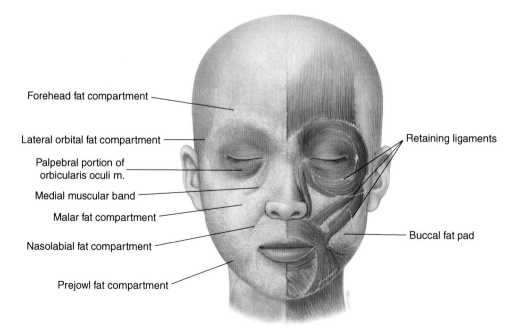

Forehead fat compartment

Lateral orbital fat compartment

Palpebral portion of orbicularis oculi m.

Medial muscular band

Malar fat compartment

Nasolabial fat compartment

Prejowl fat compartment

Retaining ligaments

Buccal fat pad

Fig. 1.3 Superficial fat and superficial muscles of the face (Published with kind permission of © Kwan-Hyun Youn 2016. All rights reserved)

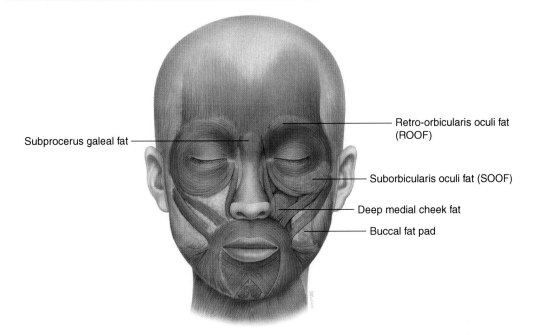

Fig. 1.4 Deep fat compartments of the face (Published with kind permission of © Kwan-Hyun Youn 2016. All rights reserved)

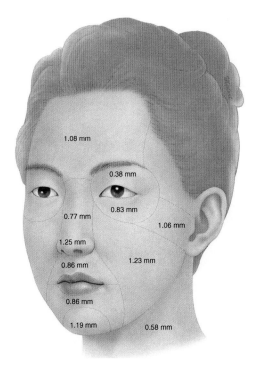

Fig. 1.5 Average skin thickness of the face (Published with kind permission of © Kwan-Hyun Youn 2016. All rights reserved)

1.3 Muscles of Facial Expressions and Their Actions

Facial mm. are attached to the facial skeleton, or membranous superficial fascia, beneath the skin, or subcutaneous tissue. The topography of the facial m. varies between males and females and between individuals of the same gender. It is important to define muscle shapes, their associations with the skin, and their relative muscular actions in order to explain the unique expressions people can make.

The face divides into nine distinct areas: (1) the forehead including glabella from eyelids to hair line, (2) temple or temporal region anterior to the auricles, (3) orbital region, (4) nose region, (5) zygomatic region, (6) perioral region and lips, (7) cheek, (8) jaws, and (9) auricle.

These muscles are distributed in different locations and (1) direct the openings of the orifices as dilators or sphincters and (2) form various facial expressions. These facial muscles, located within the superficial fascia, or subcutaneous tissue layers, originate from the facial bone or fascia and attach to the facial skin. They reveal various expressions such as sadness, anger, joy, fear, disgust, and surprise.

Facial mm. are widely distributed in different regions of the face. However, they are generally categorized different regions such as the forehead, the orbital, the nose, and other perioral regions. The platysma m., which is involved in the movement of the perioral region, is also considered a facial muscle (Fig. 1.6).

1.3.1 Forehead Region

The occipitofrontalis m. is a large, wide muscle underlying the forehead and the occipital area. It is divided into the frontal belly of the forehead region and the occipital belly of the occipital region. Clinically, the frontal belly of the occipitofrontalis m. is referred to as the "frontalis muscle" and arises from the galea aponeurosis and inserts into the orbicularis oculi m. and the frontal skin above the eyebrow. The width and contraction of the frontalis m. vary between individuals; during an individual's anxiety and surprise, this muscle produces transverse wrinkles on the forehead.

The frontalis m. is rectangular and possesses bilateral symmetry. Its muscle fibers are vertically oriented and join the orbicularis oculi and the corrugator supercilii m. near the superciliary arch of the frontal bone. The frontalis m. lies beneath the skin of the forehead (3–5 mm in average), though depth can differ considerably (27 mm) between individuals (Fig. 1.7).

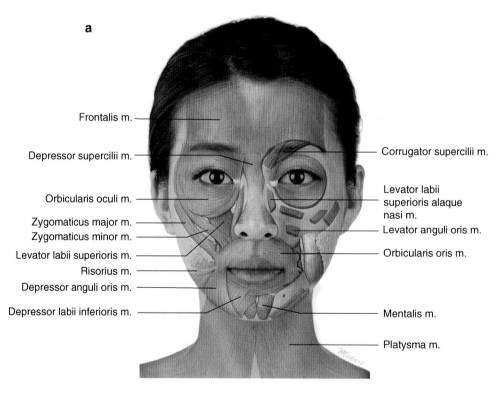

Fig. 1.6 Facial muscles. (**a**) Frontal view, (**b**) lateral view, (**c**) oblique view (Published with kind permission of © Kwan-Hyun Youn 2016. All rights reserved)

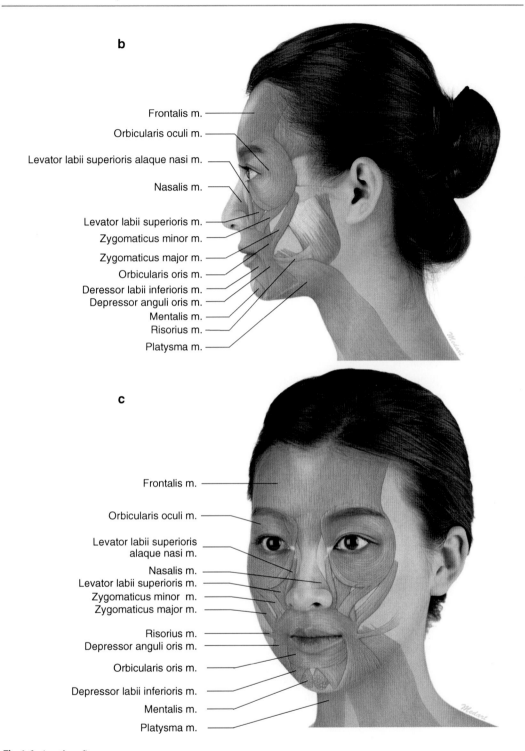

b

Frontalis m. ————
Orbicularis oculi m. ————
Levator labii superioris alaque nasi m. ————
Nasalis m. ————
Levator labii superioris m. ————
Zygomaticus minor m. ————
Zygomaticus major m. ————
Orbicularis oris m. ————
Deressor labii inferioris m. ————
Depressor anguli oris m. ————
Mentalis m. ————
Risorius m. ————
Platysma m. ————

c

Frontalis m. ————
Orbicularis oculi m. ————
Levator labii superioris alaque nasi m. ————
Nasalis m. ————
Levator labii superioris m. ————
Zygomaticus minor m. ————
Zygomaticus major m. ————
Risorius m. ————
Depressor anguli oris m. ————
Orbicularis oris m. ————
Depressor labii inferioris m. ————
Mentalis m. ————
Platysma m. ————

Fig. 1.6 (continued)

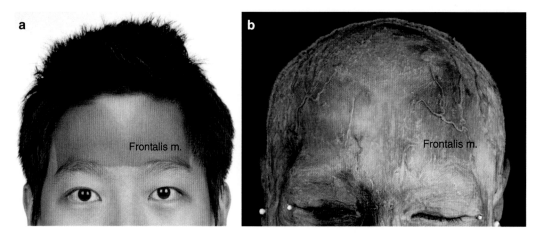

Fig. 1.7 Frontalis muscle of the forehead (**a, b**) (Published with kind permission of © Hee-Jin Kim and Kwan-Hyun Youn 2016. All rights reserved)

1.3.2 Temporal Region (or Temple)

The temporal region is confined within the boundary of the temporal fossa. Within the temporal fossa, a fan-shaped temporalis and its vessels and nerves occupy this concavity. The temporalis m. is divided into two layers: superficial and deep. A majority of the temporalis belong to the deep layer and arise from the broad temporal fossa, whereas the superficial layer of the temporalis m. arises from the internal aspect of the deep temporal fascia (temporalis muscle fascia). The deep temporal fascia (temporalis muscle fascia) is the tenacious fascia attached superiorly to the superior temporal line and inferiorly to the upper margin of the zygomatic arch.

Though the superficial layer of the temporalis developed in four-legged animals, the superficial layer in human seems very thin and rudimentary. All the temporalis muscle fibers converge as a tendon and attach to the tip of the coronoid process and to the anteromedial side of the mandibular ramus. The temporalis holds a flat, fan shape due to its broader origin and narrower attachment.

There is a region in which the muscle fibers transition into tendons. The upper half of the temporalis superior to the zygomatic arch is composed only of the muscle belly, and the lower half (roughly two- or three-digit widths) is occupied by a converged tendon and a part of the deep layer of the temporalis that is covered by the aponeurotic structure.

The temporalis m. is divided into three parts: anterior, middle, and posterior temporalis m. While its anterior temporalis fibers proceed almost vertically, the fibers of the posterior temporalis run almost horizontally. The main functions of the temporalis differ according to muscular orientation. A whole temporalis m. raises the mandible for mouth closing, providing tension to prevent the mouth from opening against gravity. The temporalis m. is innervated by the anterior, middle, and posterior deep temporal nerves from the mandibular n. It is supplied by the anterior and posterior deep temporal arteries for the anterior 2/3 of the temporalis and by the middle temporal a. for the posterior 1/3 region as well (Figs. 1.8 and 3.26).

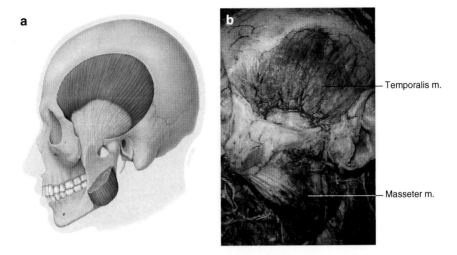

Fig. 1.8 Temporalis muscle of the temporal region (**a**, **b**) (Published with kind permission of © Hee-Jin Kim and Kwan-Hyun Youn 2016. All rights reserved)

1.3.3   Orbital Region

The shape of the eyes is well framed by moving muscles that surround it, which determine basic facial expressions. Orbicularis oculi m. is a broad, flat, elliptical muscle composed of an orbital part and a palpebral part. The palpebral part is then divided again into a superficial portion (ciliary bundle) and a deep portion (lacrimal part).

The main function of the orbicularis oculi m. is to mediate eye closure. The orbicularis oculi m. has many neighboring muscles (e.g., corrugator supercilii m., procerus m., frontalis m., zygomaticus major m., and zygomaticus minor m.), and various direct and indirect muscular connections exist between the orbicularis oculi m. and the surrounding musculature. These connections may participate in the formation of various facial expressions. In Asians, the lateral muscular band and the medial muscular band of the orbital portion of the orbicularis oculi m. are observed in 54 % and 66 % of the cases, respectively (Figs. 1.9, 1.10, 2.4, and 2.5). Furthermore, it is observed that 89 % of Asians possess direct muscular connections between the zygomaticus minor m. and the orbicularis oculi m.

The corrugator supercilii m. originates from the periosteum of the frontal bone on the medial side of the superciliary arch, proceeds superiorly and laterally, and then merges with the frontalis m. It consists of two distinct bellies—the transverse and oblique belly. The origin of the transverse belly of the corrugator supercilii m. is superior and more lateral than the origin of the oblique belly, and most of them attach to the frontalis m. (Fig. 1.11) and to the superolateral orbital part of the orbicularis oculi m. The transverse belly is located deeper and proceeds in a more horizontal direction than the oblique belly. This muscle makes narrow, vertical wrinkles on the glabellar region and presents an aged appearance by producing these wrinkles with the frontalis m.

The depressor supercilii m. is a fan-shaped or triangular-shaped muscle that originates from the frontal process of the maxilla and from the nasal portion of the frontal bone above the medial palpebral ligament. The depressor supercilii m. proceeds through the glabellar region while being mixed with the corrugator supercilii m., and it intermingles with medial fibers of the orbicularis oculi m. (Fig. 1.10).

Fig. 1.9 Orbicularis oculi muscle of the orbital region. (**a**) Frontal view, (**b**) lateral view (Published with kind permission of © Kwan-Hyun Youn and Byung-Heon Kim 2016. All rights reserved)

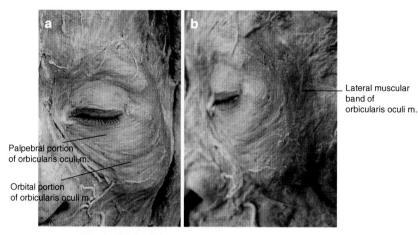

Lateral muscular band of orbicularis oculi m.

Palpebral portion of orbicularis oculi m.

Orbital portion of orbicularis oculi m.

Fig. 1.10 Medial muscular band of the orbicularis oculi muscle and upper lip elevators (Published with kind permission of © Hee-Jin Kim 2016. All rights reserved)

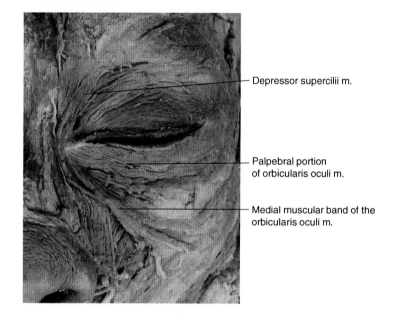

Depressor supercilii m.

Palpebral portion of orbicularis oculi m.

Medial muscular band of the orbicularis oculi m.

Oblique band of the corrugator supercilii m.   Transverse band of the corrugator supercilii m.

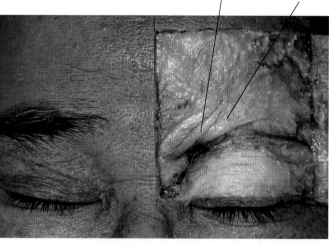

Fig. 1.11 Corrugator supercilii muscle (Published with kind permission of © Hee-Jin Kim 2016. All rights reserved)

1.3.4 Nose Region

The nose is a dynamic structure that moves nasal cartilages and plays an important role in the nasal physiology. Muscles of the nose and the nose region contain of the procerus m., the nasalis m., and the depressor septi nasi m., along with several other muscles attached to the nasal ala.

The procerus m. is a small muscle that originates from the nasal bone, proceeds superiorly, and attaches to the skin of the radix. Fibers of the frontalis m. at the insertion point are cross-locked. This muscle makes a horizontal line on the radix below the glabella by pulling the medial side of the eyebrow down (Fig. 1.12).

The nasalis consists of a transverse part and an alar part. The transverse part is a C-shaped, triangular muscle raised from the maxilla and the canine fossa to the nasal ala. The transverse part extends from the superficial layer of the levator labii superioris alaeque nasi m. The alar part is a small rectangular muscle arising from the maxilla superior to the maxillary lateral incisor and inserting into the deep skin layer of the alar facial crease of the alar cartilage. The transverse part compresses and decreases the size of the naris, while the alar part serves to enlarge the size of the naris (Fig. 1.13).

The depressor septi nasi m. is located on the deep part of the lip. This muscle arises from the incisive fossa (between the central and lateral incisors) and inserts into the moving part of the nasal septum. It pulls the nose tip inferiorly to enlarge the size of the naris (Fig. 1.12).

Furthermore, it was observed that all of the LLSAN m., 90 % of the LLS m., and 28 % of the additional fibers of the zygomaticus minor m. were attached to the nasal ala.

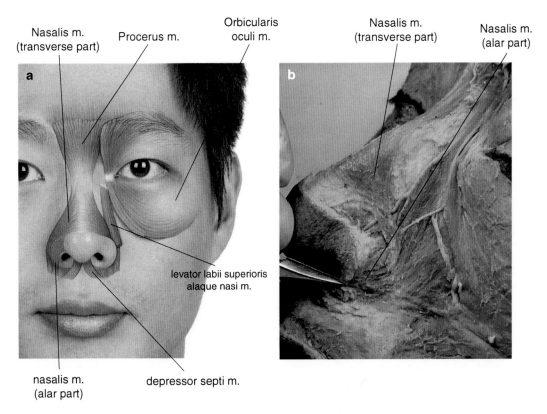

Fig. 1.12 Perinasal muscles (**a, b**) (Published with kind permission of © Hee-Jin Kim and Kwan-Hyun Youn 2016. All rights reserved)

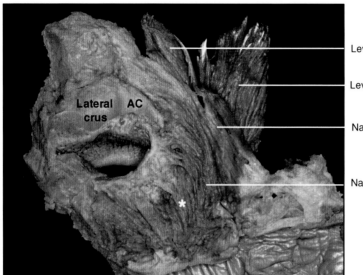

Levator labii superioris alaeque nasi m.

Levator labii superioris

Nasalis m. (transverse part)

Nasalis m. (alar part)

Fig. 1.13 The alar part of the nasalis in the posterior aspect (left side of the specimen). The N-alar is located anterior to the transverse part of the nasalis and is inserted into the alar facial crease and its adjacent deep surface of the external alar skin (*AC* accessory alar cartilage, * point between the alar facial crease and the alar groove) (Published with kind permission of © Hee-Jin Kim and Kwan-Hyun Youn 2016. All rights reserved)

1.3.5 Perioral Muscles

1.3.5.1 Intrinsic Muscles of the Lip and Cheek (Fig. 1.14)

Orbicularis Oris Muscle (OOr)
The orbicularis oris m. is a mouth constrictor surrounding the mouth region. Most muscle fibers are continuations from various muscles in the mouth region. Intrinsic orbicularis oris muscle fibers originate from the alveolar bone of the maxillary and mandibular incisors. This muscle works to close the mouth and pucker the lips.

Buccinator Muscle
The buccinator m. originates from the lateral side of the alveolar portion of maxillary and mandibular molars and from the anterior border of the pterygomandibular raphe. The buccinators consist of four bands: the first band (the superior band) originating from the maxilla, the second band originating from pterygomandibular raphe, the third band originating from the mandible, and the fourth band (the inferior band) originating inferiorly to the third band, extending inferiorly, and medially proceeding inferiorly to the orbicularis oris muscle fibers. The inferior band, unlike other bands, continues bilaterally to the median plane of the mandible (Fig. 1.15).

1.3.5.2 Dilators of the Lips

Muscles Inserted into the Modiolus
Zygomaticus Major Muscle (ZMj)
The zygomaticus major m. originates from the facial side of the zygomatic bone, proceeds inferiorly and medially, joins the orbicularis oris m., and attaches to the modiolus. Thus, the well-known function of the ZMj is elevating the mouth corner. However, the insertion pattern varies, and the fiber running deeper than the levator anguli oris m. is always observed. These fibers insert into the anterior region of the buccinators (Fig. 1.16).

Levator Anguli Oris Muscle (LAO)
The levator anguli oris m. originates from the canine fossa inferior to the infraorbital foramen, joins the orbicularis oris m., and attaches to the modiolus. It serves to elevate the mouth corner (Figs. 1.16 and 1.17).

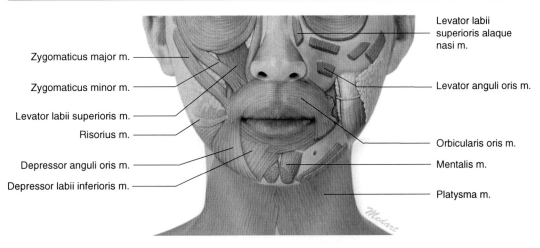

Fig. 1.14 Perioral muscles (Published with kind permission of © Kwan-Hyun Youn 2016. All rights reserved)

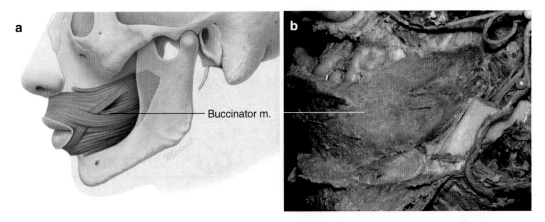

Fig. 1.15 Buccinator muscle (depressor anguli oris muscle (DAO) is reflected superiorly to show the mandibular portion attachment at the buccinators) (**a**, **b**) (Published with kind permission of © Hee-Jin Kim and Kwan-Hyun Youn 2016. All rights reserved)

Depressor Anguli Oris Muscle (DAO)
The depressor anguli oris m. is a triangular muscle that is on the most superficial layer of the perioral m. along with the risorius m. It arises from the oblique line of the mandible and merges with the depressor labii inferioris m. at the origin. This muscle becomes more narrow, proceeds to the mouth corner (modiolus), and merges with the risorius m (Fig. 1.17).

Risorius Muscle
The risorius m. is a thin and slender muscle. This muscle is predominantly located 20–50 mm lateral to the mouth corner and 0–15 mm below the inter-cheilion horizontal line. Most fibers originate from the superficial musculoaponeurotic system (SMAS), the parotid fascia, and the masseteric fascia. It sometimes also originates from the platysma m. Its fibers insert into the modiolus and pull the mouth corner when smiling (Fig. 1.18).

Muscles Inserting into the Upper and Lower Lip Between the Labial Commissure and the Midline

Levator Labii Superioris Muscle (LLS)
The levator labii superioris m. originates from 8 to 10 mm inferior to the infraorbital margin of the

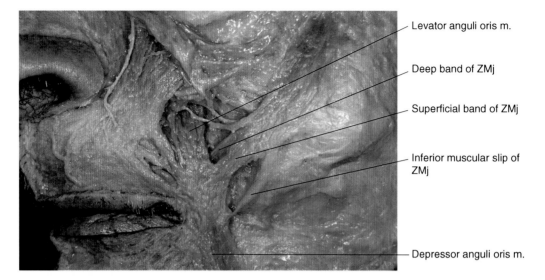

Levator anguli oris m.

Deep band of ZMj

Superficial band of ZMj

Inferior muscular slip of ZMj

Depressor anguli oris m.

Fig. 1.16 Zygomaticus major muscle (ZMj) inserting to the modiolar region. ZMj is divided into the superficial and deep band. Deep band of the ZMj is inserted to the anterior border of the buccinators which is deep inside the levator anguli oris muscle. In this photograph, inferior muscular slip of the ZMj is shown (bifid ZMj) which inserts into the depressor anguli oris (Published with kind permission of © Hee-Jin Kim and Kwan-Hyun Youn 2016. All rights reserved)

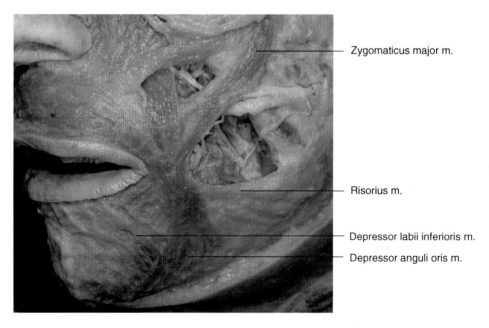

Zygomaticus major m.

Risorius m.

Depressor labii inferioris m.
Depressor anguli oris m.

Fig. 1.17 Depressor anguli oris muscle (Published with kind permission of © Hee-Jin Kim 2016. All rights reserved)

maxilla and inserts into the lateral side of the upper lip. The levator labii superioris m. is rectangular shaped rather than triangular shaped, and its medial fibers are attached to the deep side of the alar facial crease. Also, 90 % of the muscle is mixed with the alar part of the nasalis m. A part of the deep tissue of the levator labii superioris m. extends to the skin of the nasal vestibule (Figs. 1.19 and 4.34).

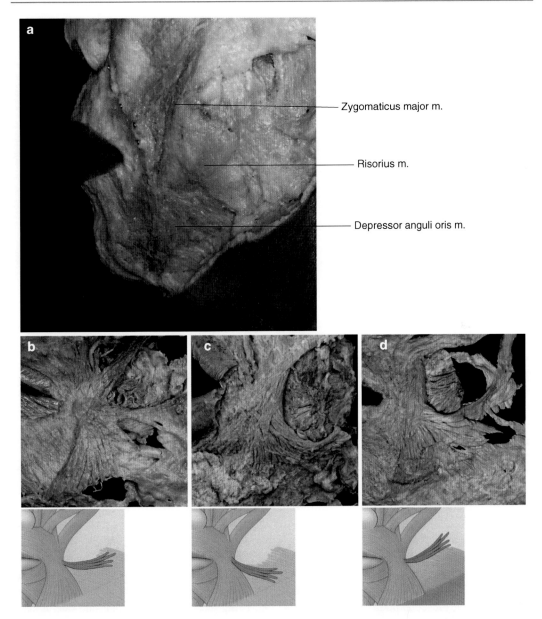

Zygomaticus major m.

Risorius m.

Depressor anguli oris m.

Fig. 1.18 Risorius muscles. (**a**) Three patterns of the risorius muscle, (**b**) platysma-risorius, (**c**) triangularis-risorius, (**d**) zygomaticus-risorius (Published with kind permission of © Hee-Jin Kim and Kwan-Hyun Youn 2016. All rights reserved)

Levator Labii Superioris Alaeque Nasi Muscle (LLSAN)

The levator labii superioris alaeque nasi m. originates from the frontal process of the maxilla and inserts into the upper lip and the nasal ala. The levator labii superioris alaeque nasi m. is divided into superficial and deep layers. The superficial layer proceeds inferiorly to the surface layer of the levator labii superioris m., and the deep layer proceeds even deeper than the levator labii superioris m. The deep and superficial layer of the levator labii superioris m. originates from the frontal process of the maxilla and inserts between the levator anguli oris and the orbicularis oris m. (Fig. 1.19).

Fig. 1.19   Major upper lip elevators. This muscle group includes the levator labii superioris alaeque nasi (*LLSAN*), levator labii superioris (*LLS*), and zygomaticus minor (*ZMi*) muscles (Published with kind permission of © Hee-Jin Kim 2016. All rights reserved)

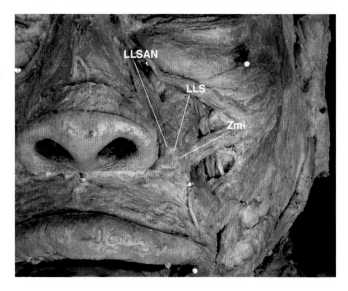

Modiolus

The modiolus is a fibromuscular structure that decussates between the orbicularis oris m. and the dilators of the lips ending at the lateral border of the cheilion. The modiolus m. lies either superior or inferior to the intercheilion line. It is strongly associated with facial expression, beauty, aging, and formation of the nasolabial fold. In Asians, the modiolus lies 11.0 ± 2.6 mm lateral, 8.9 ± 2.8 mm inferior to the cheilion, and inferior to the intercheilion line. These characteristics are mostly common in Asians, differing from Caucasians whose modiolus lies on or is superior to the intercheilion line.

Muscles that terminate at the modiolus implement formations of subtle and detailed facial expressions. The modiolus m. is a dense, compact, and mobile muscular node formed by a convergence of muscle fibers from the zygomaticus major, the depressor anguli oris, risorius, the orbicularis oris, buccinators, and the levator anguli oris. In 21.4% of Koreans, the modiolus showed tendinous tissue instead of muscular tissue as described above, and this area of convergence consisted of dense, irregular, and collagenous connective tissue (Fig. 2.33).

Zygomaticus Minor Muscle (Zmi)

The zygomaticus minor m. originates from the zygomatic bone and inserts into the upper lip. In Korean cases, 28% showed additional fibers inserting into the nasal ala in addition to the upper lip (Figs. 1.19 and 2.26).

Depressor Labii Inferioris Muscle (DLI)

The depressor labii inferioris m. originates from the oblique line of the mandible and inserts into the lower lip (Figs. 1.17 and 1.20).

Upper Lip Elevators (Fig. 1.19)

The shape of the upper lip is directed by upper lip elevators, which consist of the levator labii superioris alaeque nasi, the levator labii superioris, and the zygomaticus minor m. These muscles are used to elevate the upper lip and create smiling or sad facial expressions. Upper lip elevators are categorized into two layers with the levator labii superioris alaeque nasi m. and the zygomaticus minor m. being located on the medial and lateral side, respectively, and partially or completely covering the levator labii superioris, which is located on a deeper layer. These three muscles are localized on the lateral side of the nasal ala. Upper lip elevators are attached to the surface of the orbicularis oris m. and are involved to form the nasolabial fold.

Contracting Muscle of the Chin
Mentalis Muscle

The mentalis m. elevates the chin and the lower lip and provides major vertical support for the lower lip. Resection of the mentalis m. may cause the patient to drool and may affect the denture

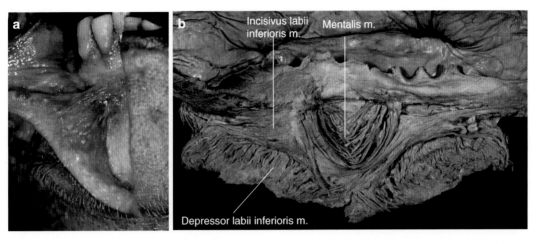

Fig. 1.20 Mentalis muscle after removal of the mandible. (**a**) Anterior aspect. (**b**) Posterior aspect (Published with kind permission of © Hee-Jin Kim 2016. All rights reserved)

Fig. 1.21 The layers of the perioral musculature (*yellow* first layer, *blue* second layer, *pink* third layer, *purple* fourth layer) (Published with kind permission of © Kwan-Hyun Youn 2016. All rights reserved)

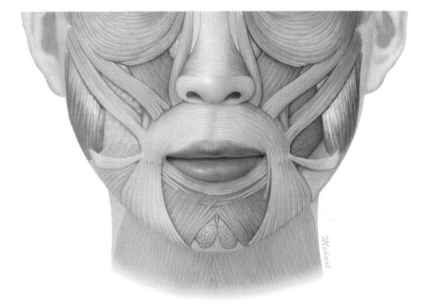

stability. This muscle is cone shaped with its apex originating from the incisive fossa of the mandible. Its medial fibers descend anteromedially and cross together, forming a dome-shaped pattern. Contraction of the mentalis m. produces a wrinkle in the skin of the mentum (Fig. 1.20).

Layers of the Perioral Muscles

The perioral m. is categorized into four layers according to depth, which is then further specified into three superficial layers and one deep layer (Fig. 1.21).

Superficial Layer

First layer

Depressor anguli oris, risorius, superficial layer of the orbicularis oris m., and superficial layer of the zygomaticus major m.

Second layer

Platysma, zygomaticus minor, and levator labii superioris alaeque nasi

Third layer

Levator labii superioris, deep layer of the orbicularis oris m., and deep layer of the depressor labii inferioris m.

Deep Layer
Fourth layer
Levator anguli oris, mentalis, deep layer of the zygomaticus major m., and buccinator

1.3.6 Platysma Muscle

The platysma m. attaches to the lower border of the mandible and to the mandibular septum and also merges with the facial m. around the lower lip. It consists of two types of fibers. A flattened bundle passes superomedially to the lateral border

of the depressor anguli oris, and the other type remains deep into the depressor anguli oris and reappears at its medial border. Lack of decussation creates a cervical defect, resulting in an elasticity reduction in the cervical skin and giving rise to the so-called gobbler neck deformity with age (Fig. 2.41). Asians experience fewer cases than Caucasians of lacking decussation, which then leads to fewer cases of the "gobbler neck." Platysmal fibers do not merely decussate but also sometimes show cases of interlacing from each side or of one side of the muscle overlapping and covering the other side (Figs. 1.22 and 1.23).

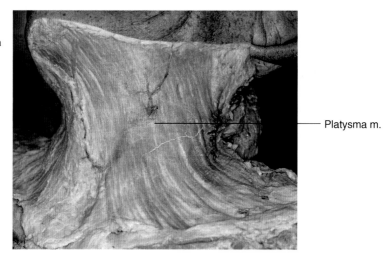

Fig. 1.22 Platysma muscle of the superficial cervical region (Published with kind permission of © Hee-Jin Kim 2016. All rights reserved)

Platysma m.

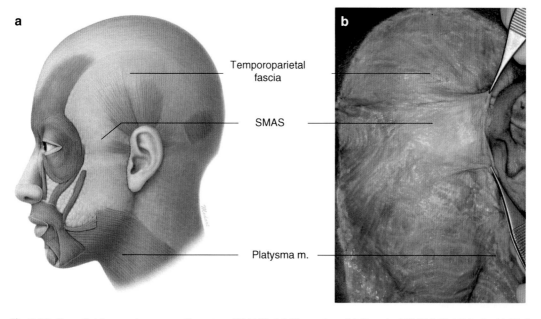

Temporoparietal fascia

SMAS

Platysma m.

Fig. 1.23 Superficial musculoaponeurotic system (SMAS). (**a**) Illustration. (**b**) Stretched SMAS (Published with kind permission of © Hee-Jin Kim and Kwan-Hyun Youn 2016. All rights reserved)

1.4   SMAS Layer and Ligaments of the Face

The superficial musculoaponeurotic system (SMAS) is a continuous fibromuscular layer investing and interlinking the muscles of facial expression. It has been found to consist of three distinct layers: a fascial layer superficial to the musculature, a layer intimately associated with the mimic m., and a deep layer extensively attached to the periosteum of the bones of the face. In addition to its usefulness as a deep layer to tighten during an aging face surgery, it serves as a guide to the depth of key neurovascular structures.

The face, like other body parts, also has several ligament structures, which firmly supports surrounding tissues. This retaining ligament is broadly and firmly attached from the periosteum, or fascia, to the dermis. These strong retaining ligaments in the face can be divided into true (osteocutaneous) and false (fasciocutaneous) ligaments according to its strength, attachment, and function.

The true retaining ligament originates from the periosteum, attaches to the dermis, and gives strong support to the soft tissue. True retaining ligaments consist of the orbicularis retaining ligament, the zygomatic ligament, the zygomatic cutaneous ligament, the lateral orbital thickening, the mandibular ligament, etc.

There are multiple false retaining ligament attachments that exist at sequential facial planes. These attachments emanate from the dermis and attach to the underlying SMAS, but it does not retain strongly. The false retaining ligaments are particularly strong over the forehead, eyes, nose, lip, and chin areas. They are of intermediate strength over the lateral cheek and neck areas and tend to be relatively loose over the medial cheek and temple areas (Figs. 1.24 and 1.25). Therefore, they easily lose elasticity and sag with age, causing changes in facial features due to fat redistribution and drooping. False retaining ligaments consist of the masseteric cutaneous ligament, the platysma-auricular ligament, etc.

Superior Temporal Septum

The superior temporal septum's fascia adheres to the superior temporal line of the skull. This structure appears to be merging with the temporal fascia and the periosteum of the skull. This merging ends as a temporal ligamentous adhesion at the lateral third of the eyebrow and occurs 10 mm superior to the supraorbital margin with a height of 20 mm and a width of 15 mm.

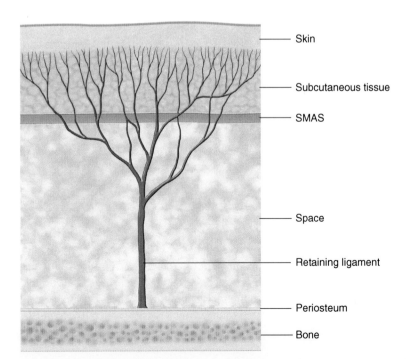

Fig. 1.24 Schematic illustration of the retaining ligament from the periosteum to the skin (Published with kind permission of © Kwan-Hyun Youn 2016. All rights reserved)

Skin

Subcutaneous tissue

SMAS

Space

Retaining ligament

Periosteum

Bone

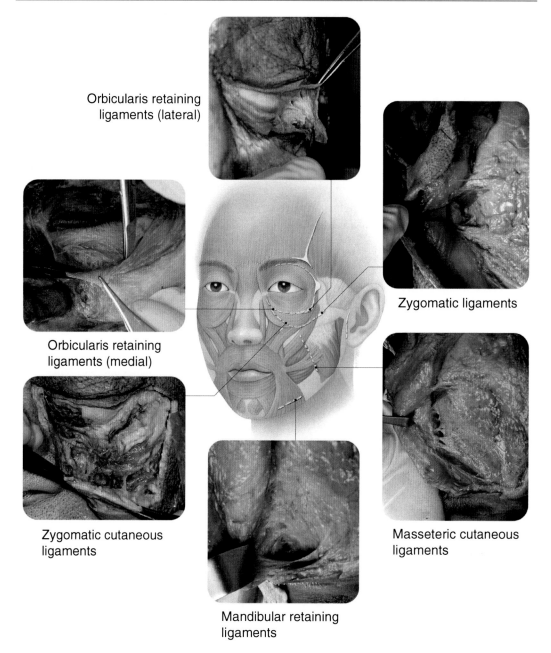

Orbicularis retaining
ligaments (lateral)

Zygomatic ligaments

Orbicularis retaining
ligaments (medial)

Zygomatic cutaneous
ligaments

Masseteric cutaneous
ligaments

Mandibular retaining
ligaments

Fig. 1.25 The retaining ligaments of the face (Published with kind permission of © Hee-Jin Kim and Kwan-Hyun Youn 2016. All rights reserved)

Zygomatic Ligament

The zygomatic ligament, also known as the McGregor's patch, is located posterior to the origin of the zygomaticus minor m. This structure is a true retaining ligament that connects the lower margin of the zygomatic arch to the skin.

Zygomatic Cutaneous Ligament

The zygomatic cutaneous ligament originates from the periosteum of the zygomatic bone, proceeds along the lower margin of the orbicularis oculi m., and attaches to the skin on the anterior portion of the zygomatic bone. The soft tissues in this area are maintained by the ligament, which droops with age in the form of a malar mound (or baggy lower eyelid).

Orbicularis Retaining Ligament
The orbicularis retaining ligament is located superiorly, inferiorly, and laterally along the orbital rim. It attaches to the lateral periosteum of the orbit and extends to the deep portion of the orbicularis oculi m.

Lateral Orbital Thickening
Lateral orbital thickening is located on the superolateral side of the orbital margin and originates from the orbital retaining ligament.

Mandibular Retaining Ligament
The mandibular retaining ligament connects the periosteum of the mandible, located right underneath the origin of the depressor anguli oris m., to the skin.

Masseteric Cutaneous Ligament
The masseteric cutaneous ligament is a false retaining ligament originating from the anterior

border of the masseter m. This ligament attaches to the SMAS and to the skin covering the cheek. It attenuates with age and causes the SMAS to sag and jowl.

Platysma-Auricular Fascia (PAF)
The platysma-auricular fascia is a compact fibrous tissue located inferior to the ear lobule where the lateral temporal-cheek fat compartment and the postauricular fat compartment merge.

1.5   Nerves of the Face and Their Distributions

The trigeminal n. and the facial n. are major nerves distributed on the face. The trigeminal n. consists of three parts: the ophthalmic n., the maxillary n., and the mandibular n. The trigeminal n. passes through the foramina of the skull and divides into independent facial sensory nerves (Fig. 1.26). On the other hand, the facial n. has one nerve trunk that passes through the stylomastoid foramen and separates into two divisions

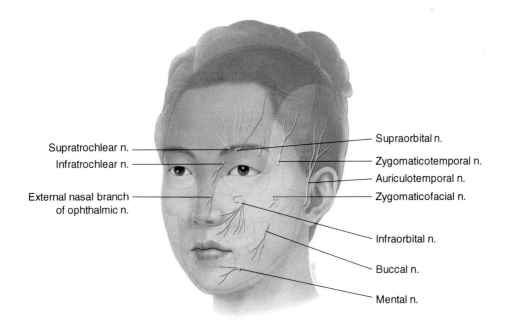

Fig. 1.26 The cutaneous sensory distribution of the face (*red zone* area of the ophthalmic nerve (V1) branches, *yellow zone* area of the maxillary nerve (V2) branches, *green zone* area of the mandibular nerve (V3) branches) (Published with kind permission of © Kwan-Hyun Youn 2016. All rights reserved)

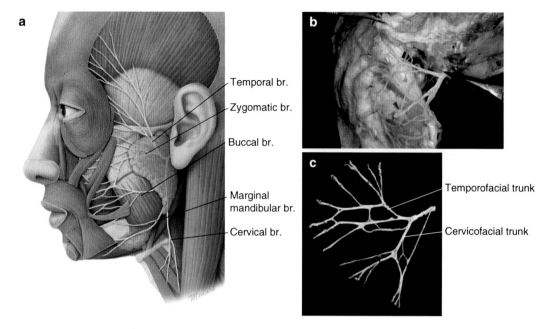

Fig. 1.27 Trunk of the facial nerve (**a, b, c**) and its temporofacial (*upper*) and cervicofacial (*lower*) divisions (Published with kind permission of © Hee-Jin Kim and Kwan-Hyun Youn 2016. All rights reserved)

(temporofacial and cervicofacial divisions) within the parotid gland. Later, it branches off into five different nerve bundles transmitting motor impulses to facial mm. (Fig. 1.27).

1.5.1   Distribution of the Sensory Nerve

Supraorbital n., supratrochlear n. (ophthalmic n.): forehead, glabellar region
Infratrochlear n. (ophthalmic n.): glabella, radix
Infraorbital n. (maxillary n.): external nose, nasal septum, lower eyelid, upper lip
Buccal n. (mandibular n.): cheek, cheilion
Mental n. (mandibular n.): lower lip, mentum, cheilion

1.5.2   Distribution of the Motor Nerve

The facial n. consists of temporal, zygomatic, buccal, marginal mandibular, and cervical nerve branches that transmit motor impulse to facial

and neck muscles. There are several small nerve branches with complicated, random distribution patterns to the muscles. Therefore, it is difficult to determine nerve distribution region of boundaries for each muscle (Fig. 1.27).

1.5.3   Upper Face

1.5.3.1 Distribution of the Sensory Nerve

The upper face includes the forehead, the glabella, the radix, and the upper and lower eyelids. The supraorbital n. distributes to the forehead, the glabella, and the upper eyelid with its long, distinct branch and runs to the forehead and the glabellar region. Furthermore, the minor branches of the supraorbital n. distribute to the upper eyelid in a triangular pattern. The supratrochlear n. is distributed to the upper eyelid and the medial side of the glabella. The inferior palpebral branch of the infraorbital n. moves superiorly past the infraorbital foramen and is distributed to the lower eyelid in a triangular pattern. Also, several minor branches of the zygomaticofacial n. become distributed to the inferior and medial side of the lower eyelid.

1.5.3.2 Distribution of the Motor Nerve

The temporal branch of the facial n. moves super-omedially toward the upper eyelid and is distributed to the muscles on the lateral side of the upper eyelid. The zygomatic branch of the facial n. distributes the orbit and the muscles on the lateral side of the lower eyelid as it runs superior to the inferior palpebral branch of the infraorbital n. Generally, the temporal branch transmits motor ability to the frontalis m., the corrugator supercilii m., and the superior portion of the orbicularis oculi. The zygomatic branch is distributed to the inferior portion of the orbicularis oculi m. and to the origins of the zygomaticus major and minor m.

Typically, the buccal branch of the facial n. runs superiorly along the lateral side of the nose to the radix. Therefore, the procerus m., the medial portion of the corrugator supercilii m. on the glabella, and the radix are innervated by the temporal branch and by the buccal branch (Figs. 1.28 and 1.29).

1.5.4 Midface

1.5.4.1 Distribution of the Sensory Nerve

The midface includes the cheek region and the nose. The infraorbital n. of the trigeminal n. plays a vital role in the cutaneous sensation in the midface. The external nose is mostly innervated by the infraorbital n. with the exception of some parts that are innervated by the external nasal branch of the nasociliary n. (from ophthalmic n.). The lateral nasal branch of the infraorbital n. proceeds along the nasal ala with some distributing to the nose tip near the midline. The internal nasal branch of the infraorbital n. is distributed to the mucosal of the nasal septum. The superior labial branch of the infraorbital n., one of the most distinct branches, is distributed to the area that spans from the medial portion of the upper lip to the cheilion. The infraorbital n. is distributed among the general infraorbital region from the infraorbital foramen to the upper lip.

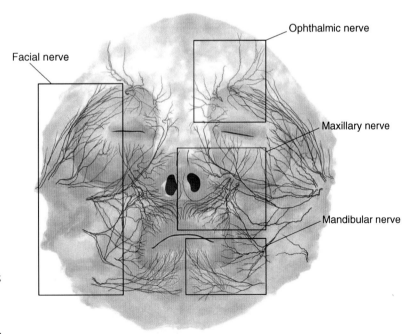

Fig. 1.28 Sensory and motor nerve distribution on the face (V1, ophthalmic nerve; V2, maxillary nerve; V3, mandibular nerve; VII, facial nerve) (Published with kind permission of © Kwan-Hyun Youn 2016. All rights reserved)

a

b

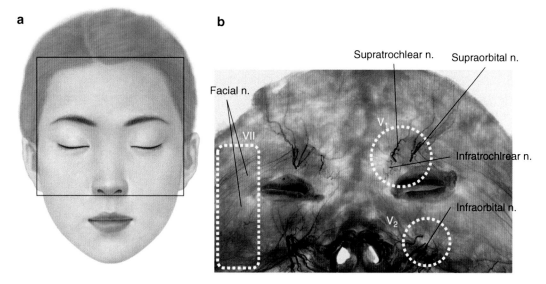

Supratrochlear n.   Supraorbital n.

Facial n.

VII

V_1

Infratrochlrear n.

Infraorbital n.

V_2

Fig. 1.29 Sensory and motor nerve distribution at the forehead and periorbital region. This specimen was prepared to show the intramuscular nerve distribution by Sihler's technique (V1, ophthalmic nerve; V2, maxillary nerve; VII, facial nerve) (**a**, **b**) (Published with kind permission of © Hee-Jin Kim and Kwan-Hyun Youn 2016. All rights reserved)

1.5.4.2 Distribution of the Motor Nerve

The buccal branch of the facial n. proceeds medially and has small branches that are dispersed to the cheek. These branches superimpose with the superior labial branch of the infraorbital n. The buccal branch and the infraorbital n. lie superimposed with each other in the superior 3/4 of the infraorbital region. The buccal branch is distributed to the levator labii superioris alaeque nasi, the levator labii superioris, and the zygomaticus minor m. The buccal branch also is distributed to the zygomaticus major, the risorius, and the superior portion of the orbicularis oris m. (Figs. 1.28 and 1.30).

1.5.5 Lower Face

1.5.5.1 Distribution of the Sensory Nerve

In the lower face, the mandibular n. distributes to the lower lip and to the mentum. The buccal n. proceeds medially along the occlusal plane to the cheilion. The mental n. runs through the mental foramen and is distributed to the lower lip which includes the cheilion and the mandible. The supe-

rior labial branch of the infraorbital n., the buccal n., and the angular branch of the mental n. is distributed to the mouth corner. Furthermore, there are nerve plexus formed between the infraorbital n. and the buccal n. and also between the buccal n. and the mental n. superior and inferior to the cheilion.

1.5.5.2 Distribution of the Motor Nerve

The marginal mandibular branch of the facial n. is distributed to the mentalis, the depressor anguli oris, the depressor labii inferioris, and the inferior portion of the orbicularis oris m. The actual anatomy of the trigeminal n. and the facial n. is quite different from that found in the textbook. The cutaneous n. of the trigeminal n. and the motor n. of the facial n. are not distinguished as some of the few, distinct nerves. Even though some of the major branches can be observed during dissection surgeries with the naked eye, they are intertwined with other small branches such as nets. Therefore, it is best to describe the distribution pattern of nerves with a plane rather than with several distinct lines (Figs. 1.28 and 1.31).

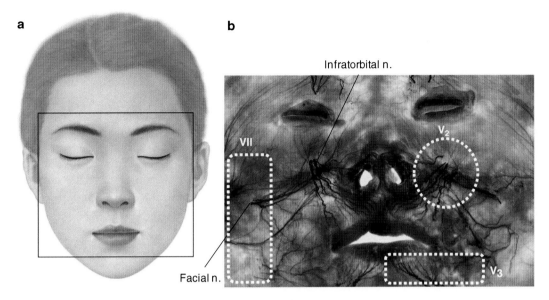

Fig. 1.30 Sensory and motor nerve distribution at the midfacial region. This specimen was prepared to show the intramuscular nerve distribution by Sihler's technique (V2, maxillary nerve; V3, mandibular nerve; VII, facial nerve) (**a, b**) (Published with kind permission of © Hee-Jin Kim and Kwan-Hyun Youn 2016. All rights reserved)

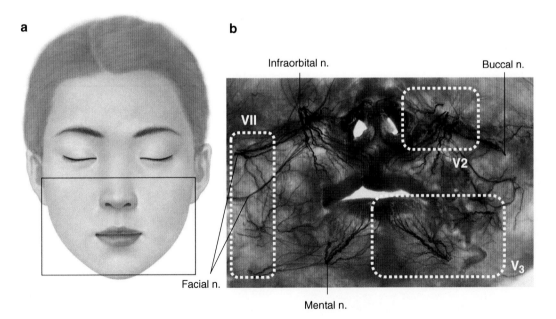

Fig. 1.31 Sensory and motor nerve distribution at the perioral and lower face region. This specimen was prepared to show the intramuscular nerve distribution by Sihler's technique (V2, maxillary nerve; V3, mandibular nerve; VII, facial nerve) (**a, b**) (Published with kind permission of © Hee-Jin Kim and Kwan-Hyun Youn 2016. All rights reserved)

1.6 Nerve Block

1.6.1 Supraorbital Nerve Block (SON Block)

The supraorbital n. originates from the supraorbital notch, which can be identified on the supraorbital rim. If the supraorbital notch cannot be found externally, it can be replaced by the supraorbital foramen. The supraorbital notch is located medial to the mid-pupillary line on the frontal bone. Insert the syringe immediately inferior to the eyebrow and inject anesthetics proximal to the supraorbital notch. It is necessary to take caution to avoid injecting the anesthetics into the orbit. If the lateral branch has not been anesthetized with a general infraorbital nerve block, it is suggested to perform additional anesthesia by inserting the syringe 1 cm superior to the orbit toward the medial portion of the eyebrow (Fig. 1.32).

1.6.2 Supratrochlear Nerve Block (STN Block)

In 30 % of cases, the supratrochlear n. arises together with the supraorbital n. from the supra-

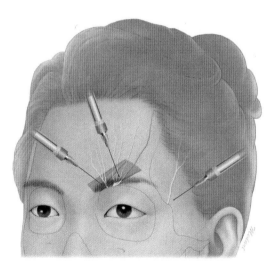

Fig. 1.32 Supraorbital and supratrochlear nerve block (Published with kind permission of © Kwan-Hyun Youn 2016. All rights reserved)

orbital notch and can perform nerve blocks along with SON blocks. However, in the majority of cases (70 %), the supratrochlear n. originates separately from the frontal notch, which requires an injection 15 mm lateral from the facial midline, which can be approximated by placing the index finger on the midline of the forehead. In this case, an additional injection is required (Fig. 1.32).

1.6.3 Infraorbital Nerve Block (ION Block)

The infraorbital nerve block is an extremely useful technique to use in aesthetic surgery procedures as both intraoral and extraoral approaches could perform effectively. Both approaches target the infraorbital foramen, which the infraorbital n. passes. The infraorbital foramen is located on the upper third where the line between the nasal ala superior to the vertical line passing the cheilion and the point at the same height as the infrabital margin is divided into three sections (Figs. 1.33 and 1.49).

In the extraoral approach, inject anesthetics targeting the location of the infraorbital foramen as described above. However, the transcutaneous, nasolabial approach of approaching from the marionette line rather than by vertical insertion also exists. This approach injects at the site where the superior portion of the marionette line and the alar groove meet to form the upside-down V-shape and then runs superolaterally. The transcutaneous nasolabial method allows for a more intricate approach to the infraorbital foramen (Fig. 1.33a).

In the intraoral approach, place the syringe parallel to the longer axis of the maxillary second premolar and inject the needle slowly and superiorly. Inject anesthetics when the target is located (Fig. 1.33b). Both approaches require caution to avoid injecting the anesthetic inside of the orbit. In such cases, diplopia may occur.

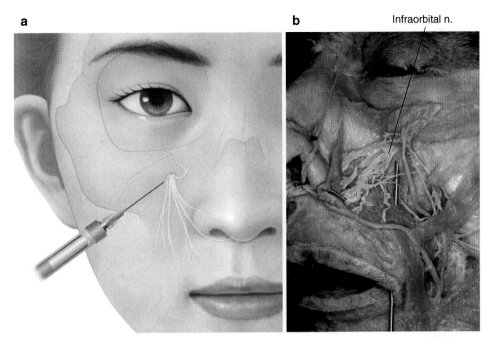

Fig. 1.33 Extraoral (**a**) and intraoral (**b**) approaches for the infraorbital nerve block (Published with kind permission of © Hee-Jin Kim and Kwan-Hyun Youn 2016. All rights reserved)

1.6.4   Zygomaticotemporal Nerve Block (ZTN Block)

The meeting point of the frontal bone and the zygomatic bone is presented as an eminence point lateral to the eyebrow. The zygomaticotemporal n. originates laterally to this region and innervates the lateral portion of the eyebrow and the glabellar region. However, facial landmarks are unclear. Therefore, a nerve block does not always perform well (Fig. 1.32).

1.6.5   Mental Nerve Block (MN Block)

Similar to the infraorbital nerve block, a mental nerve block can also be completed via the extraoral or the intraoral approach. Both approaches target the mental foramen 2 cm vertically inferior from the cheilion. For the extraoral approach, inject the syringe posterior to and superomedially while targeting the mental foramen (Fig. 1.34a, c).

In the intraoral approach, inject slowly, inferiorly, and posteriorly at the mandibular second premolar region (Fig. 1.34b, c).

1.6.6   Buccal Nerve Block (BN Block)

The buccal nerve enters the oral mucosa near the maxillary second molar, its main trunk running medially. As it proceeds medially through the dentition, the main trunk of the buccal n. lies in a slightly inferior position. The main trunk of the buccal n. supplies the entire buccal area including the mucosa and skin of the lateral area of the mouth corner. The main trunk gives off some branches not only near the main trunk running inferomedially, but also in the other regions. The buccal nerve block should be performed with a needle approaching the buccal aspect of the mandibular second molar. After placing a needle parallel to the occlusal plane, inject the anesthetic slowly along the buccal aspect of the mandibular second molar or oblique line of the mandible (Fig. 1.35).

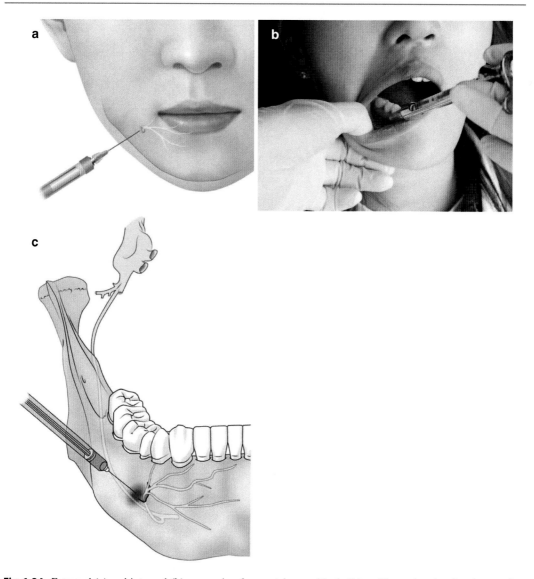

Fig. 1.34 Extraoral (**a**) and intraoral (**b**) approaches for mental nerve block ((**c**) an illustration showing the anesthetized area) (Published with kind permission of © Hee-Jin Kim and Kwan-Hyun Youn 2016. All rights reserved)

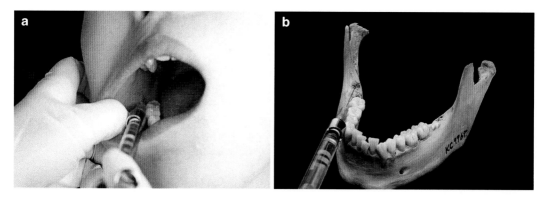

Fig. 1.35 Buccal nerve block (**a, b**) (Published with kind permission of © Hee-Jin Kim 2016. All rights reserved)

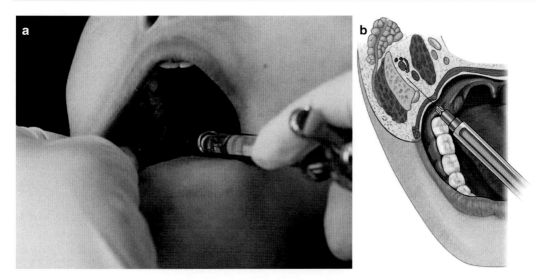

Fig. 1.36 Inferior alveolar nerve block (**a, b**) (Published with kind permission of © Hee-Jin Kim and Kwan-Hyun Youn 2016. All rights reserved)

1.6.7 Inferior Alveolar Nerve Block (IAN Block)

In order to completely anesthetize the skin on the lower chin, it is necessary to intraorally approach the inferior alveolar n. Slowly inject a long needle 1 cm superior to the occlusal plane of the first premolar on the opposite side of the target toward the central point on the retromolar triangle. If the needle comes into contact with the ramus of the mandible, pull it back slightly and inject anesthetics (Fig. 1.36).

1.6.8 Auriculotemporal Nerve Block (ATN Block)

For an auriculotemporal nerve block, inject 2 cc of anesthetics anterior to the tragus. If the auriculotemporal n. is blocked, the sensation of the tragus, the anterior auricle, and the external auditory meatus also become blocked. Anesthetizing other parts of the auricle requires a great auricular nerve block (Fig. 1.37).

1.6.9 Great Auricular Nerve Block (GAN Block)

The great auricular n. proceeds superiorly along the anterior surface of the sternocleidomastoid m. Place a hand on the patient's temple in order to distinguish the sternocleidomastoid m. and mark its boundary. Then inject the anesthetic 6.5 cm along the line from the external acoustic pore to the midpoint between the boundaries of the sternocleidomastoid m. (Fig. 1.37).

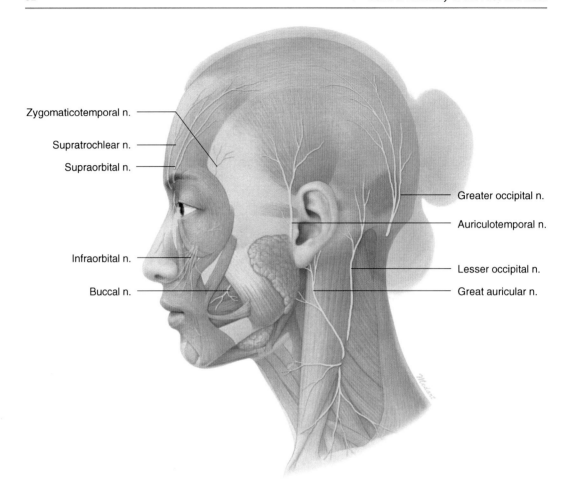

Zygomaticotemporal n.

Supratrochlear n.

Supraorbital n.

Greater occipital n.

Auriculotemporal n.

Infraorbital n.

Lesser occipital n.

Buccal n.

Great auricular n.

Fig. 1.37 Topographic anatomy of peripheral sensory nerve branches of the head and neck (Published with kind permission of © Kwan-Hyun Youn 2016. All rights reserved)

1.7   Facial Vessels and Their Distribution Patterns

Facial blood vessels are extremely important. As filler injections become more common, blood vessel-related issues, such as skin necrosis and blindness, will become more prominent. Therefore, more in-depth studies on blood vessel pathways in terms of injection techniques are required.

Clinically, facial blood vessels do not follow one specific pattern. Dissections show many variations of this pattern. Furthermore, facial blood vessels contain not only arteries but also veins

and their branches. It is impossible to perfectly avoid every single blood vessel during blind injections. However, with enough knowledge of these vessels, it is possible to minimize risks and perform a safe injection.

Chapter 1 deals with general and typical patterns of the facial a., and Chaps. 3, 4, and 5 describes patterns, depths, and variations of vessel types that branch according to their regions and their clinical significances.

The blood supply of the head and neck is mostly given by the common carotid a. The right common carotid a. and the right subclavian a. are arising from the brachiocephalic trunk. On the other side, the left common carotid a. and the left subclavian a. are arising independently from the aortic arch. At the level of the superior border of the thyroid cartilage, the common carotid a. divides into internal and external carotid arteries. The pulse of the common carotid a. can be felt when touching the anterior border of the sternocleidomastoid m. at the level of the thyroid cartilage.

The internal carotid artery has no other arterial branches except the ophthalmic a. before reaching the brain. The internal carotid a. runs anteromedially through the carotid canal and enters the middle cranial fossa. The internal carotid a. supplies blood to the cerebrum, and a portion enters the orbit area, arrives at the superomedial side of the orbital, and supplies blood to the eye, the orbit, and the lacrimal gland.

The external carotid a. originates from the common carotid a. in the area of the carotid sheath. Although the origin of the external carotid a. lies anteriorly and medially from the internal carotid a., it locates further laterally as it ascends. This artery divides into eight branches.

The facial blood supply is given by the internal carotid a. and the external carotid a. These arteries are accompanied by the corresponding sensory n. On the superficial layer of the skin, branches of the external carotid a. (facial a., superficial temporal a., facial branches of the maxillary a.) and branches of the internal carotid a. (supraorbital a. branching from the ophthalmic a., supratrochlear a., infratrochlear a.) supply blood to this layer (Figs. 1.38 and 1.39).

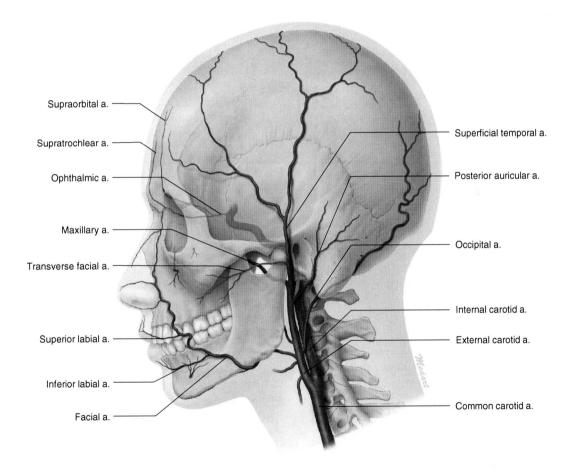

Fig. 1.38 External and internal carotid arterial system and their branches (Published with kind permission of © Kwan-Hyun Youn 2016. All rights reserved)

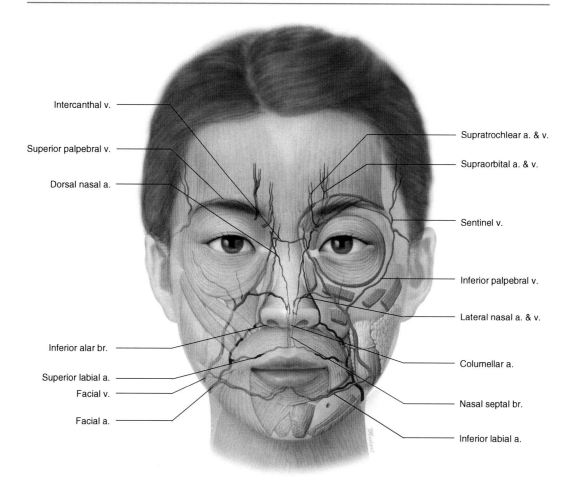

Intercanthal v.

Superior palpebral v.

Dorsal nasal a.

Supratrochlear a. & v.

Supraorbital a. & v.

Sentinel v.

Inferior palpebral v.

Lateral nasal a. & v.

Inferior alar br.

Superior labial a.

Facial v.

Facial a.

Columellar a.

Nasal septal br.

Inferior labial a.

Fig. 1.39 General courses and locations of the artery and vein on the face (Published with kind permission of © Kwan-Hyun Youn 2016. All rights reserved)

1.7.1 Facial Branches of the Ophthalmic Artery (Fig. 1.40)

1.7.1.1 Supraorbital Artery
The supraorbital a., together with the supraorbital n., originates from the supraorbital notch, or the supraorbital foramen, and supplies the upper eyelid, forehead, and the scalp region.

1.7.1.2 Supratrochlear Artery
The supratrochlear a. runs more medially than the supraorbital artery and supplies the upper eyelid, the forehead, and the scalp.

1.7.1.3 Dorsal Nasal Artery
The dorsal nasal a. originates from the medial canthus of the orbit together with the infratrochlear n. and supplies the medial portion of the upper eyelid, the lacrimal sac, and the dorsum of the nose.

1.7.1.4 Lacrimal Artery
The lacrimal a. is the last, small part of the ophthalmic a. that originates from the lateral side of the supraorbital margin and supplies the lateral side of the upper eyelid.

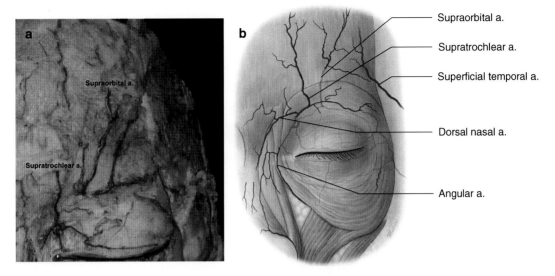

Fig. 1.40 Periorbital arterial distribution of the ophthalmic artery (internal carotid arterial system) (**a**, **b**) (Published with kind permission of © Hee-Jin Kim and Kwan-Hyun Youn 2016. All rights reserved)

1.7.1.5 External Nasal Artery
The external nasal a. runs through the junction between the nasal bone and the nasal cartilage. It supplies the intermediate zone of the external nose inferior to the nasal bone.

1.7.2 Facial Branches of the Maxillary Artery
(Fig. 1.41)

1.7.2.1 Infraorbital Artery
The infraorbital a. exits the infraorbital foramen inferior to the orbit and branches to the inferior palpebral branch, the nasal branch, and the superior labial branch.

1.7.2.2 Zygomatic Artery
Two branches of the zygomatic a. (zygomaticofacial branch and zygomaticotemporal branch) pass along the zygomatic canal on the lateral wall of the orbit. The zygomaticofacial branch exits the zygomaticofacial foramen and supplies the zygomatic region and the cutaneous layer of the cheek. The zygomaticotemporal branch exits the zygomaticotemporal foramen

and supplies the cutaneous layer of the temporal region.

1.7.2.3 Buccal Artery
The buccal a. runs to the muscle internally between the ramus of the mandible and the masseter m. It branches to the surface of the cheek and supplies the cutaneous and mucosal layer of the cheek and the molar gingiva on the buccal side.

1.7.2.4 Mental Artery
The mental a. branches from the inferior alveolar a. inside the mandibular canal. It exits the mental foramen along with the mental n. and supplies the chin, the lower lip, and the mandibular incisive gingiva.

1.7.3 Facial Artery

The facial a. branches from the external carotid a., winds through the antegonial notch, passes the masseter m. anteriorly, and runs tortuously to the nasion and the glabella. It is known that the facial a., which runs superomedially through the face, branches to the inferior labial a., the superior

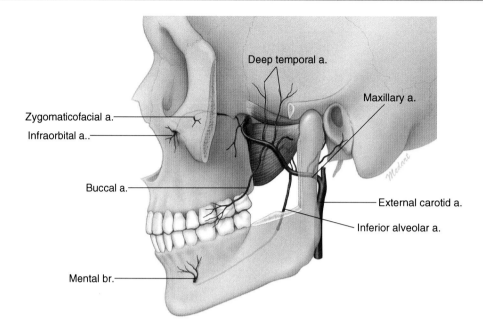

Fig. 1.41 Maxillary artery and its branches (Published with kind permission of © Kwan-Hyun Youn 2016. All rights reserved)

labial a., and the lateral nasal a. and terminates as the angular a. (Fig. 1.42). The facial a. is described in many textbooks as running from the mandibular angle to the radix and is in charge of most of the blood supply to the face. The facial a. continues all the way to the angular a. in only 36.3 % cases among 91 Korean hemifaces. In other races, the angular a. was observed in 4 % of French hemi-faces, 12 % of Japanese hemi-faces, 22 % of Turkish hemi-faces, and 68 % of British hemi-faces. Although the research presented differences of angular a. occurrences among various ethnicities, the actual cause for that difference is still unclear, because the fractions of populations observed to possess angular a. were quite different between French and British populations despite both of them being Caucasian. What is quite apparent, however, is the fact that general documentation stating that the facial a. proceeds to the angle of the orbit seems erroneous (Fig. 1.42).

Facial a. symmetry is observed in only 30 % of the cases, and regions with sparse blood supply are supplied additionally by branches of the superficial temporal a. (transverse facial a.,

supraorbital a., supratrochlear a.), branches of the ophthalmic a., and branches of the maxillary a. (infraorbital a., mental a.). The more prominent arteries on the opposite side of the face can also supply these regions.

1.7.3.1 Facial Artery Branches

Superior, Inferior Labial Branch
The facial a. proceeds obliquely and superiorly to the angle of the mouth, and branches of the superior labial a. to the upper lip and branches of the inferior labial artery to the lower lip appear.

Inferior Alar Branch
The inferior alar branch divides off from the facial a. immediately adjacent to the nasal ala and runs to the columella. It merges with columellar branches from the superior labial a. and forms an artery that runs through the columella all the way to the nasal tip.

Lateral Nasal Branch
The lateral nasal branch supplies the nasal ala and the nasal bridge, divides lateral to the nasal

Fig. 1.42 General concept about the course of the facial artery. This concept is controversial according to many studies of the facial artery (Published with kind permission of © Kwan-Hyun Youn 2016. All rights reserved)

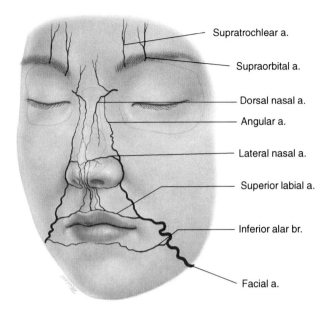

- Supratrochlear a.
- Supraorbital a.
- Dorsal nasal a.
- Angular a.
- Lateral nasal a.
- Superior labial a.
- Inferior alar br.
- Facial a.

ala, and runs along the lateral side of the nose. It continues to the nasal branch of the infraorbital a. and the external nasal branch of the ophthalmic a.

Angular Artery

The angular a. is the terminal artery of the facial a. after it branches from the lateral nasal and runs superiorly to the canthus. It terminates at the medial canthus region and branches to the medial side of the eyelid and the nose. The angular a. sometimes branches from the ophthalmic branch rather than from the facial a., but it is observed to be the terminating branch of the facial a. in 51 % of the cases.

1.7.3.2 Typical Distribution Patterns of the Facial Artery

Branches of the facial a. are categorized into four types depending on their directions, locations, and supplying regions (lower lip, upper lip, nasal, and infraorbital region). The branching pattern can be generally organized into three categories depending on the region: type I (nasolabial pattern; 51.8%), type II (nasolabial pattern with infraorbital trunk; 29.6%), and type III (forehead pattern; 18.6%) (Fig. 1.43).

1.7.4 Frontal Branch of the Superficial Temporal Artery

The superficial temporal a. is the terminal branch of the external carotid a. that emerges from the facial side between the temporomandibular joint and the ear and runs superiorly to the scalp. It branches to the transverse facial a. immediately inferior to the ear and is located about 2 cm inferior to the zygomatic arch. The superficial temporal a. branches to both the frontal branch and the parietal branch 37 mm superior and 18 mm anterior from the tragus. The frontal branch runs obliquely toward the forehead and has either one branch (94.8%) or two branches (5.2%) that approach the frontalis m. past its lateral border and supply the region (Fig. 1.44). The superficial temporal a. passes the lateral side of the head along with auriculotemporal n. It branches to the transverse facial a. approximately 1 cm inferior to the zygomatic arch, runs superiorly, and divides into the frontal branch, which supplies the lateral side of the forehead, and into the parietal branch, which supplies the parietal region. The transverse facial a. runs anteriorly, merges with the branch

Fig. 1.43 Three patterns of the facial artery (FA). (**a**) *Type I* nasolabial pattern, (**b**) *type II* nasolabial pattern with infraorbital trunk, (**c**) *type III* forehead pattern (*Ag* angular a., *LN* lateral nasal a., *IA* inferior alar br., *SL* superior labial a., *IL* inferior labial a., *FA* facial a.) (Published with kind permission of © Kwan-Hyun Youn 2016. All rights reserved)

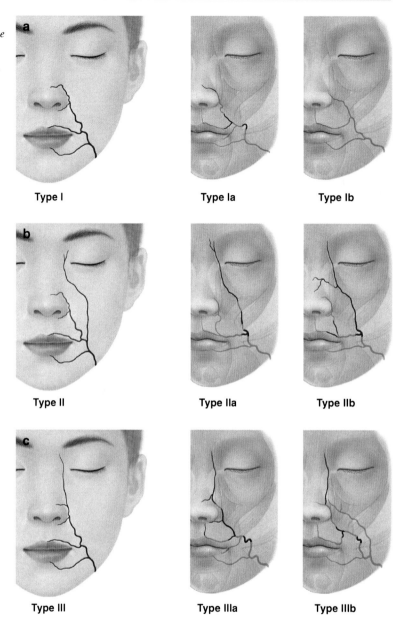

Type I   Type Ia   Type Ib

Type II   Type IIa   Type IIb

Type III   Type IIIa   Type IIIb

of the facial a., and supplies the parotid gland and the cheek.

1.7.5   Facial Veins

The facial v. follows the same distribution pattern as the facial a. with a few differences. Typically, the facial v. presents a greater amount of pattern variation than the facial a. (Fig. 1.45).

1.7.5.1 Veins with Cutaneous Nerves and Arteries

The facial v. runs in the direction opposite from the corresponding facial a. Veins of the forehead, the scalp, and the upper eyelid run to the superior ophthalmic v. on the orbit. The veins of the upper lip, the lateral side of the nose, and the lower eyelid run through the infraorbital v. to the infratemporal region and the pterygoid plexus.

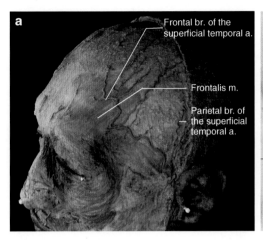
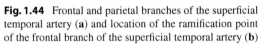
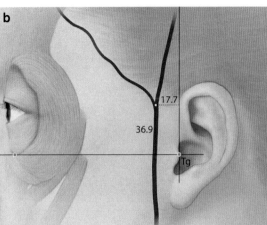

Fig. 1.44 Frontal and parietal branches of the superficial temporal artery (**a**) and location of the ramification point of the frontal branch of the superficial temporal artery (**b**)

1.7.5.2 Facial Vein

The facial v. parallels the facial a. in most instances. However, it runs more posteriorly than the facial a. and is less tortuous in the opposite direction of the facial a. The facial v. branches as follows (Fig. 1.45).

Angular Vein

The angular v. is formed through the merging of the supraorbital v. and the supratrochlear v. at the canthus. The angular v. branches into two different branches with one flowing into the orbit and continuing to the superior ophthalmic v. and the other proceeding superficially and running inferiorly along the face as a facial v (Fig. 1.46a).

Intercanthal Vein

The intercanthal v. has been observed at the glabella and the radix in 71 % of the cases and is located along the midpupillary line on the subcutaneous layer. 63.4 % of the cases showed that the intercanthal v. was observed along the line connecting the bilateral canthus, and the other 7.3 % of the cases showed that the vein was observed inferior to the same line. All the observed intercanthal veins run through the more superficial subcutaneous layer rather than the procerus m. (Figs. 1.46b and 1.47).

Facial Vein

The facial v. obliquely runs posteroinferiorly toward the mandibular angle, receiving many tributaries.

External Nasal Vein

The external nasal v. originates from the lateral side of the nose and connects to branches of the infraorbital v.

Deep Facial Vein

The deep facial v. connects to the pterygoid plexus in the deep layer of the face.

Labial Vein

The labial v. originates from the upper lip and the lower lip. The superior labial v. connects to the infraorbital v. The inferior labial v. connects to the mental v. The facial v. continues inferiorly along the antegonial notch toward the neck. The facial v., unlike the facial a., runs through the superficial portion of the mandible.

1.7.5.3 Retromandibular Vein

The superficial temporal v. runs inferiorly, merging with the branch from the parotid gland and exits the lower margin of the parotid gland. The retromandibular v. is bifurcated into the anterior and posterior branch at the mandibular angle.

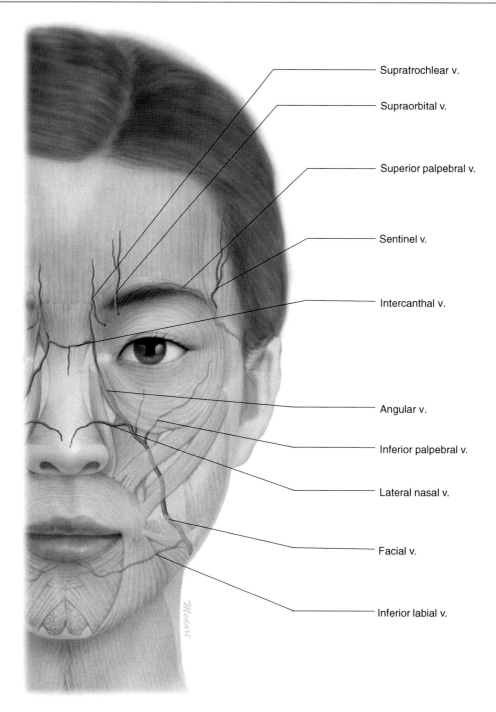

Supratrochlear v.

Supraorbital v.

Superior palpebral v.

Sentinel v.

Intercanthal v.

Angular v.

Inferior palpebral v.

Lateral nasal v.

Facial v.

Inferior labial v.

Fig. 1.45 General course of the facial vein and its topographic relationships with the facial muscles (Published with kind permission of © Kwan-Hyun Youn 2016. All rights reserved)

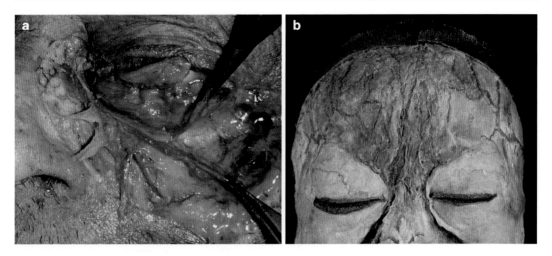

Fig. 1.46 Veins at the medial canthal region (**a**) and radix and glabella (**b**) (Published with kind permission of © Hee-Jin Kim 2016. All rights reserved)

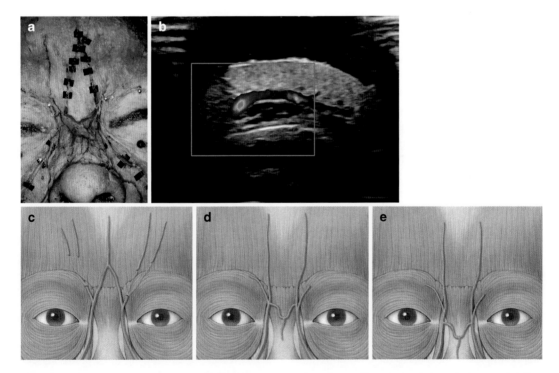

Fig. 1.47 Venous anastomoses (intercanthal vein) at the glabellar region. (**a**) Intercanthal vein (ICV) is located within the subcutaneous tissue at the radix and glabella (sonography, **b**), and ICVs are classified into three patterns based on its location ((**c**) type I at the glabellar region, (**d**) type IIa at the level above the intercanthal line, (**e**) type IIb at the level below the intercanthal line) (Published with kind permission of © Hee-Jin Kim and Kwan-Hyun Youn 2016. All rights reserved)

The posterior branch merges with the posterior auricular v. from the posterior portion of the ear and forms the external jugular v.

The anterior branch of the retromandibular v. merges with the facial v. at the neck and forms the common facial v. The common facial v. continues into the internal jugular v.

1.7.5.4 Superficial Temporal Vein
The superficial temporal v. receives the vein branch from the lateral side of the head. It proceeds inferiorly along the anterior side of the ear and enters the parotid gland. The superficial temporal v. merges with the maxillary v. from the inferior portion of the temporal region inside the parotid gland.

1.7.6 Connections of the Vein

The facial v. lacks valves and is connected to relatively fewer branches. These two following vein connections are extremely important.

1.7.6.1 Connection Between Facial Vein and Angular Vein
The facial v. passes the angular v. and connects directly to the superior ophthalmic v. The venous blood from the medial canthus flows through the facial v. inferiorly to the neck or through the superior ophthalmic v. to the orbit. The superior ophthalmic v. proceeds into the cavernous sinus with a slow blood flow rate.

1.7.6.2 Connection Between the Pterygoid Plexus and the Cavernous Sinus
The venous blood from the facial v. flows through the deep facial v. again and into the pterygoid plexus inferior to the temporal region. The pterygoid plexus connects to the cavernous sinus inside the skull.

1.8 Facial and Skull Surface Landmarks

1. 44 Facial Surface Landmarks According to Anatomical Labels (Fig. 1.48)
2. Surface Landmarks of the Skull
   It is best to be acquainted with foramens of the skull, which serve as landmarks from which major vessels and nerves exit.
   (a) The frontal notch and the supraorbital foramen: The frontal notch medial to the eye could feel near the glabella along the supraorbital margin, and the supraorbital foramen could feel slightly lateral to the frontal notch. The supratrochlear a. and supratrochlear n. pass through the frontal notch, and the supraorbital a. and supraorbital n. pass through the supraorbital foramen.
   (b) Infraorbital foramen: The infraorbital foramen is located on the upper third of the line connecting the infraorbital margin to the nasal ala. The infraorbital foramen locates medial to the vertical line connecting the pupil and mental foramen. The infraorbital a. and infraorbital n. exit through the infraorbital foramen (Fig. 1.49).
   (c) Mental foramen: The mental foramen is located along the same line used to locate the infraorbital foramen 2 cm inferior to the oral commissure. The mental n. exits through the mental foramen (Fig. 1.49).
3. Surface Anatomy (Fig. 1.50)
4. Actions of the Facial Muscles and Formation of Creases (Fig. 1.51)
   There are various muscles in the face that participate in the formation of facial expressions and facial creases. The following three points should be considered.

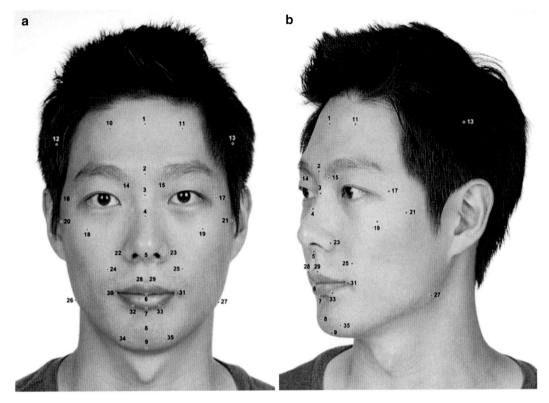

Fig. 1.48 Surface landmarks of the face ((**a**) frontal view, (**b**) oblique view) (Published with kind permission of © You-Jin Choi 2016. All rights reserved)

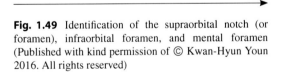

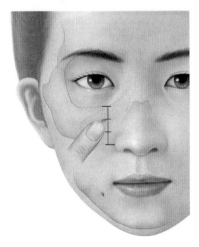

Fig. 1.49 Identification of the supraorbital notch (or foramen), infraorbital foramen, and mental foramen (Published with kind permission of © Kwan-Hyun Youn 2016. All rights reserved)

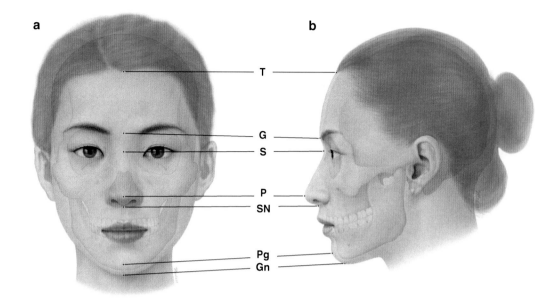

Fig. 1.50 Major anatomical landmarks of the face ((**a**) frontal view, (**b**) lateral view) (*T* trichion (hairline), *G* glabella (most anterior projection of the forehead), *S* sellion (the deepest point of the nasofrontal concavity), *P* pronasale (apex nasi, nasal tip), *SN* subnasale (the point at which the nasal septum merges), *Pg* pogonion (the most prominent point of the soft tissue of chin), *Gn* gnathion (the lowest part of the soft tissue of the chin)) (Published with kind permission of © Kwan-Hyun Youn 2016. All rights reserved)

1. First, there are origin and insertion points for the facial m., and the muscle contracts toward the origin in order to produce facial expressions and creases. Therefore, it is necessary to understand each muscle's movement vectors and their actions.
2. Second, all the wrinkles or furrows are created perpendicularly to the muscle vectors.
3. Third, there are many instances when multiple muscles overlap. Furthermore, multiple muscles are involved in producing one's facial expressions. Therefore, each muscle's movements cannot be correlated to one facial expression.
4. Fourth, not all muscles lie on the same plane. There are about 3–4 layers of depth with different muscles in each layer, which affect injection depth.

Muscle size and location vary among individuals. For example, some possess a thicker corrugator supercilii m., while others possess a wider depressor anguli oris m. It is necessary to observe a patient's various facial expressions in order to investigate the strength and area of each muscle.

Figure 1.51 uses arrows to depict the direction of facial m. contraction to help in understanding each muscle's movements and actions. The actions are organized in a table. Chapter 2 deals with each muscle's anatomy required for botulinum toxin injection.

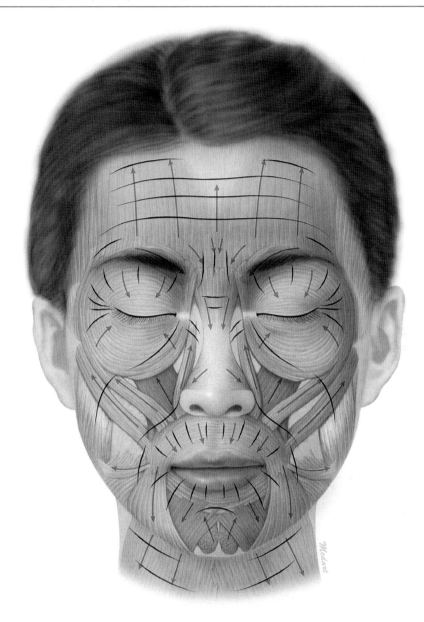

Fig. 1.51   Facial muscles and their actions (*arrows*) (Published with kind permission of © Kwan-Hyun Youn 2016. All rights reserved)

1.9   Characteristics of Asian (Korean) Skull and Face

Caucasian heads are dolichocephalic and mesocephalic shaped. However, Asians, including Koreans, show brachycephalic head shapes. Brachycephalic shaped heads indicate that the head width is relatively large in comparison to its length. Similarly, Asians possess relatively flat faces. They are particularly characterized by a protruding zygomatic bone in the anterolateral direction and a pronounced mandibular angle.

Asians also typically possess flat noses along with flat lateral facial aspects among their facial features. From their profiles, Asians possess more shallow facial depths than Caucasians (Fig. 1.52).

1. Length-breadth index: This is the ratio between the cranial length and its breadth. Asians (Koreans) typically show brachycranic (short cranium) shapes. In the females, more pronounced characteristics are shown.
2. Length-height index: This is the ratio between the cranial length and height. Both Asian genders are hypsicranic (high cranial vault) with little differences between the sexes.

3. Breadth-height index: This is the ratio between the cranial breadth and height. Asian males are typically acrocranic (high cranial vault), while females are typically metrocranic (average cranium), showing differences between genders.
4. Upper facial index: This is the ratio between the facial breadth and height and helps to identify facial morphology. Both males and females belong to the mesene face which is closer to a leptene shape (narrow face).
5. Transverse craniofacial index: This is the ratio between the cranial breadth and the facial breadth and can identify protrusions of the zygomatic bone and arch. Asian males show

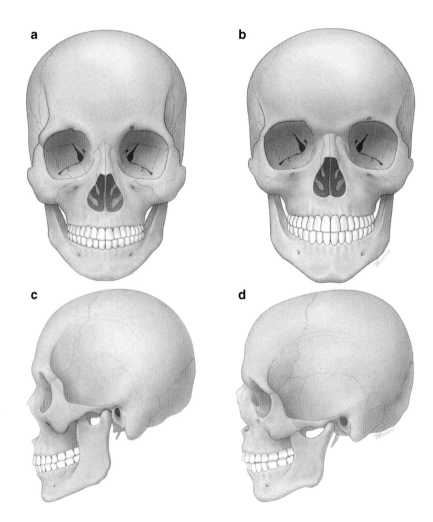

Fig. 1.52
Anthropological difference of the skull between Asian (Korean) and Caucasian ((**a, c**) Korean skull, (**b, d**) Caucasian skull) (Published with kind permission of © Kwan-Hyun Youn 2016. All rights reserved)

higher indexes, indicating that males have more pronounced zygomatic regions than females.

6. Transverse frontal index: This is an indicator for the morphology of the forehead. Asians generally show divergent morphology among females, indicating an exceptionally narrow shape.

7. Frontoparietal index: This index is the ratio between the minimum forehead breadth and the maximum head breadth and identifies the morphology of the forehead when observed from above. Both males and females show stenometopic (narrow forehead) shapes.

8. Frontozygomatic index: This index is the ratio between the forehead breadth and the zygomatic bone breadth and identifies the development of the frontal bone. Females show higher values of this index, which may indicate that they show more oval-shaped facial morphology than males.

9. Nasal index: This index is the ratio between the height of the piriform aperture and its breadth and has a varied range among Asians. Therefore, Asians (Koreans) were identified as possessing varied nasal morphology. In particular, Koreans tend to be more mesorrhine (medium sized) shaped in average.

The orbit is also one of the facial features along with the zygomatic bone that clearly indicate Korean anthropological features. According to North Korean research, Koreans are the only group to possess high orbit out of all the Asians. However, it could be verified that not many Koreans possess high hypsicinchs. Rather, the majority of Koreans were categorized as possessing mesoconch (medium orbit) traits. Furthermore, the orbital index, which compares the orbital breadth and height, indicates differences according to gender. The heights of the orbit on both sides are similar, but the orbital breadth of the right side tends to be longer. Therefore, the right orbit has a more oval shape. The orbital dimension is closely related to the development of the zygomatic bone, and interorbital breadths can be used as a criterion for determining race.

The zygomatic bone is especially pronounced in Asians and is an important anthropological feature. Zygomatic bones of Koreans were observed to have smaller angles, protrude more, and be more angular in females. In addition, the widths of the zygomatic arch in Koreans reported to be larger than Japanese and smaller than other Asian populations. The zygomatic bone is larger in males than in females and also slightly larger in the right aspect. Koreans show average-sized zygomatic bone among Asians.

The differences in dimensions between males and females are also apparent in other populations including Koreans. Generally, the dimensions of the head and face of Korean females are about 96 % the dimension of Korean males. On the other hand, the head dimensions of Caucasian females are about 90 % the dimension of Caucasian males. Therefore, the difference is much larger in Caucasians than in Koreans.

Symmetry is an important aesthetic factor. A symmetrical face is known to be more aesthetically pleasing than an asymmetric face. Asymmetry has two patterns with the right side of the face being longer than the left and with the left side of the face being wider than the right. This is the general pattern regardless of race.

When compared with Caucasians and Africans, Asians have a different shaped palpebral fissure, which determines the shape of the eye. Koreans typically have narrow and oblique palpebral fissures bulged together with the epicanthal fold. The epicanthal fold can be observed in around 57 % of the cases regardless of race.

The percentage of maximum head length of Asians in comparison to maximum head height is 80 %, which contrasts from Caucasians. The glabella lies slightly inferior to the 2/3 point of the

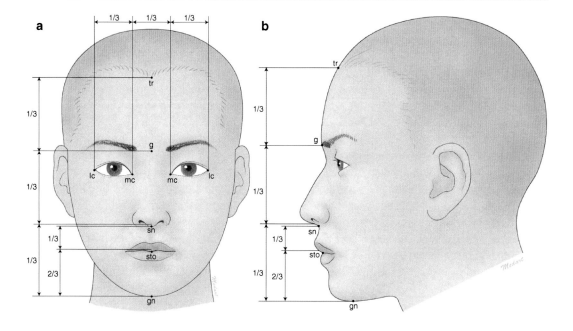

Fig. 1.53 Anthropological characteristics of the Korean face (**a, b**) (Published with kind permission of © Kwan-Hyun Youn 2016. All rights reserved)

maximum head height; the subnasale lies slightly inferior to the halfway point on the glabella; and the stomion lies inferior to the lower third of the face. Therefore, there is a tendency for Asians to show smaller, lower faces than Caucasians (Fig. 1.53).

1.10   Anatomy of the Aging Process

In life, the aging process comes naturally. Research on the aging process increased as people's average life span became longer, and people started to pay greater attention to their quality of life. Understanding the characteristics of aging is the key foundation for filler and botulinum toxin treatment (Fig. 1.54).

All tissues change characteristics with age. As apparent in Fig. 1.55, tissues are subject to atrophoderma, redistribution, and sagging. The skin loses some collagen and elastin in the dermis, and the dermis loses some hyaluronic acid, becoming dry, inelastic, and wrinkly.

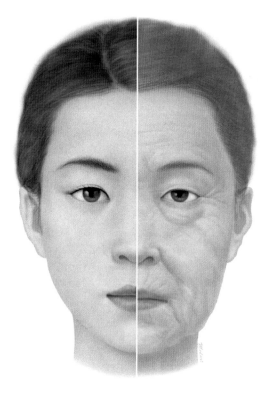

Fig. 1.54 Changes of the facial aging (Published with kind permission of © Kwan-Hyun Youn 2016. All rights reserved)

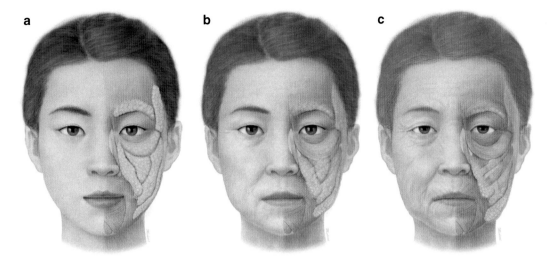

Fig. 1.55 Processes of the facial aging in 30's (**a**), 50's (**b**), and 70's (**c**) (Published with kind permission of © Kwan-Hyun Youn 2016. All rights reserved)

1.10.1 Aging Process of the Facial Tissue

The anatomical structures of the face related to aging comprise of the facial bone, fat tissue, fibrous connective tissue, and facial muscles.

The bony tissue is a structure that forms the basic frame of the face and bone remodeling goes throughout lifelong period. With aging, bone resorption is accelerated and morphologic changes take place in the marginal area of bones, such as the orbital rim, maxilla, and the mandible. Thus, the orbital rim enlarges, the maxilla shortens, and the length and height of the mandible reduce (Fig. 1.56).

Fat tissue shows different aging processes between superficial and deep fat of the face. In the superficial fat, drooping appears due to gravity. In the deep fat, relocation and atrophy take place due to the unbalanced change of the volume of fat compartments. Drooping of the fat tissues is presented as jowl or the deepening of the nasolabial fold caused by the drooping of the superficial fat of the chin and cheek. The relocation and atrophy of fat appear as hollow cheek (Fig. 1.57).

Among the fibrous connective tissue, the thick fibrous connective tissue that has high density and strongly holds facial muscle is called the retaining ligaments. The facial musculature is a thin layer that lies between the superficial fat and deep fat of the face. Fibrous connective tissue loses its elasticity when proteins such as collagen and elastin are degraded. Subsequently, dermal thickness reduces and membranous structures such as septum and SMAS shift downward.

However, retaining ligaments have two sides of aging. Retaining ligaments make the wrinkle look deeper around the boundary of the fat compartments. This is because the retaining ligaments have a function of resisting against drooping of other tissues. On the other hand, when aging proceeds and even the retaining ligament loses its elasticity, fat protrusion and drooping caused by gravity accelerate even more. An example of the former case is tear trough caused by orbicularis retaining ligament and of the latter case is palpebromalar groove and festoon caused by septal fat protrusion.

The aging of facial muscle becomes permanent through reduced elasticity of the muscle itself and through repetitive movements over a long time. A typical example of reduced muscular elasticity is the gobbler neck deformity caused by the laxity of platysma. Examples of muscle

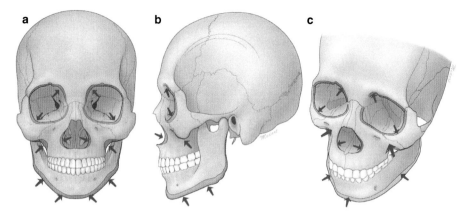

Fig. 1.56 Bone resorption pattern of the face with aging ((**a**) frontal view, (**b**) lateral view, (**c**) oblique view) (Published with kind permission of © Kwan-Hyun Youn 2016. All rights reserved)

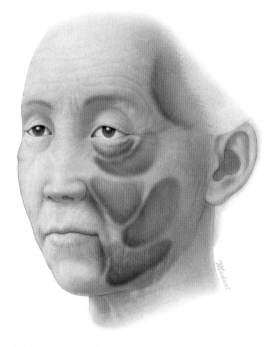

Fig. 1.57 The aging changes of the soft tissue of the face. *Brown-colored* areas indicate the remarkable volume loss with age. *Purple-colored* areas show the protrusion and drooping of the fat tissues (Published with kind permission of © Kwan-Hyun Youn 2016. All rights reserved)

fixation or adhesion with aging are deep skin wrinkles such as horizontal forehead lines, crow's feet, and horizontal upper lip line.

1.10.2 The Complex Changes of the Facial Appearance with Aging

Aging of the periorbital area progresses with a complex aging procedure of the bony orbit, orbicularis retaining ligament, superficial and deep fat, and orbicularis oculi muscle. When young, tear trough appears due to the orbicularis retaining ligament located in the medial aspect of the orbit. With age, the septal fat above the orbicularis retaining ligament goes through protrusion. Then the tear trough deepens, and margins are connected and form a nasojugal groove. The repetitive movement of the orbicularis oculi muscle at this state forms crow's feet on the lateral orbital rim. When aging further progresses, the orbital rim is absorbed and the bearing capacity, elasticity of ORL, is reduced. Consequently, festoon appears due to septal fat protrusion (Fig. 4.2).

Aging of the perioral area progresses with a complex aging procedure of the maxilla and mandible, mandibular ligament, superficial and deep fat, and perioral muscle. When young, nasolabial fold appears at the border of the upper lip and superficial malar fat compartments. As the body ages, the nasolabial fold deepens since the superficial malar fat above the nasolabial fold droops down and the cheek becomes hollow. People with active movements of DAO may form labiomandibular fold on medial boundary of DAO. The labio-mandibular fold could connect with the nasolabial fold. When aging progresses, the superficial buccal fat starts to droop and a pit appears in the mid-chin because the mandibular ligament holds the buccal fat. If the elasticity of the mandibular ligament reduces and mandible absorption accelerates the loss of support, jowling may intensify. When old, not only the mandible and maxilla are absorbed, but the alveolar bone is absorbed intensely. Since the absorption of the maxilla is faster than the mandible, the chin may seem protruded. Since the tooth and alveolar bone are lost and not there to locate the perioral muscle, the perioral muscle and lip contract and fine wrinkles appear at the perioral area.

Suggested Reading

Physical Anthropological Traits in Asians

1. Choi BY, Lee KS, Han SH, Park DK, Lim NH, Koh KS, Kim HJ, Kang HS. Group analysis using the metric measurements of Korean skulls. Korean J Phys Anthropol. 2001;14:207–15.
2. Chung MS, Kim HJ, Kang HS, Chung IH. Locational relationship of the supraorbital notch or foramen and infraorbital and mental foramina in Koreans. Acta Anat. 1995;154:162–6.
3. Ha RY, Nojima K, Adams Jr WP, Brown SA. Analysis of facial skin thickness: defining the relative thickness index. Plast Reconstr Surg. 2005;115:1769–73.
4. Han SH, Hwang YI, Lee KH, Koh KS, Choi BY, Lee HY, Sir WS, Chung MS, Kim HJ, Kim DW, Kang HS. Craniometric study in modern Korean adults. Korean J Phys Anthropol. 1995;8:205–13.
5. Hu KS, Yang SJ, Kwak HH, Park HD, Youn KH, Jung HS, Kim HJ. Location of the modiolous and the morphologic variations of the risorius and zygomaticus major muscle related to the facial expression in Koreans. Korean J Phys Anthropol. 2005;18:1–11.
6. Hwang YI, Lee KY, Choi BY, Lee KS, Sir WS, Kim HJ, Koh KS, Han SH, Chung MS, Kim H. Study on the Korean adult cranial capacity. J Korean Med Sci. 1995;10:239–42.
7. Kim HJ, Paik DJ, Choi BY, Chung MS, Han SH, Hwang YI, Sohn HJ, Chung RH, Koh KS. Measurements of the zygomatic bones and morphology of the zygomaticofacial and zygomaticotemporal foramina in Korean. Korean J Phys Anthropol. 1997;10:225–34.
8. Kim HJ, Kim KD, Choi JH, Hu KS, Oh HJ, Kang MK, Hwang YI. Differences in the metric dimensions of

craniofacial structures with aging in Korean males and females. Korean J Phys Anthropol. 1998;11:197–212.
9. Kim HJ, Lee SI, Chung IH. The morphology of the mental foramen in Korean adult mandibles. Korean J Anat. 1995;28:67–74.
10. Kim HS, Oh JH, Choi DY, Lee JG, Choi JH, Hu KS, Kim HJ. Three-dimensional courses of zygomaticofacial and zygomaticotemporal canals using Micro-CT in Korean. J Craniofac Surg. 2013;24:1565–8.
11. Kim SH, Kim NY, Lee SH, Choi HG, Shin DH, Uhm KI, Lee JY, Song WC, Koh KS. Anthropometric analysis of the mouth in Koreans. J Korean Soc Plast Reconstr Surg. 2008;35:139–46.
12. Kim SH, Whang E, Choi HG, Shin DH, Uhm KI, Chung H, Song WC, Koh KS. Analysis of the midface, focusing on the nose: an anthropometric study in young Koreans. J Craniofac Surg. 2010;21: 1941–4.
13. Kim YS, Chung MS, Park DK, Song WC, Koh KS. Asymmetric study on the Korean skull using bilateral measurements. Korean J Phys Anthropol. 2000;13: 271–9.
14. Koh KS, Han SH, Song WC, Shon HJ, Paik DJ, Kim HJ, Choi BY. Secular changes of cephalic index in Korean adults. Korean J Phys Anthropol. 2001;14: 177–85.
15. Koh KS, Hwang YI, Sohn HJ, Han SH, Paik DJ, Kim HJ, Choi BY, Lee HY, Chung MS. Re-evaluation of the orbital dimensions in modern Korean adult skulls. Korean J Phys Anthropol. 1995;8:195–204.
16. Koh KS, Shon HJ, Rhee EK, Park SJ, Kim HJ, Han SH, Chung RH. Anthropological study on the facial flatness of Korean from the historic to the modern period. Korean J phys Anthropol. 1999;12:211–21.
17. Koh KS, Song WC, Shon HJ, Kim HJ, Park DK, Han SH. The asymmetry of the nonmetric traits of Korean adult skulls. Korean J Phys Anthrop. 2000;13: 253–61.
18. Kwak HH, Park HD, Youn KH, Hu KS, Koh KS, Han SH, Kim HJ. Branching patterns of the facial nerve in Korean. Korean J Phys Anthropol. 2003;16:66–74.
19. Rho NK, Chang YY, Chao YY, Furuyama N, Huang P, Kerscher M, Kim HJ, Park JY, Peng P, Rummaneethorn P, Rzany B, Sundaram H, Wong CH, Yang Y, Prasetyo AD. Consensus recommendations for optimal augmentation of the asian face with hyaluronic acid and calcium hydroxylapatite fillers. Plast Reconstr Surg. 2015;136(5):940–56.
20. Song WC, Kim SH, Paik DJ, Han SH, Hu KS, Kim HJ, Koh KS. Location of the infra-orbital and mental foramen with reference to the soft tissue landmarks. Plast Reconstr Surg. 2007;120:1343–7.
21. Song WC, Kim SJ, Kim SH, Hu KS, Kim HJ, Koh KS. Asymmetry of the palpebral fissure and upper eyelid crease in Koreans. J Plast Reconstr Aesthet Surg. 2007;60:251–5.
22. Song WC, Park SH, Koh KS. Metric and non-metric characteristics of Korean eyes using standardized photographs. Korean J Phys Anthropol. 2002;15:95–107.

23. Yang HM, Hu KS, Kim HJ. Nervous communication and facial expression muscles. Korean J Phys Anthropol. 2013;26:1–12.

24. Youn KH, Kim YC, Hu KS, Song WC, Kim HJ, Koh KS. An art anatomical study of the facial profile of Korean. Korean J Phys Anthropol. 2002;15:251–62.

Muscles of the Face and Neck

25. Bae JH, Choi DY, Lee JG, Tansatit T, Kim HJ. The risorius muscle: anatomic considerations with reference to botulinum neurotoxin injection for masseteric hypertrophy. Dermatol Surg. 2014;40(12): 1334–9.

26. Bae JH, Lee JH, Youn KH, Hur MS, Hu KS, Tansatit T, Kim HJ. Surgical consideration of the anatomic origin of the risorius in relation to facial planes. Aesthet Surg J. 2014;34:NP43–49.

27. Choi DY, Kim JS, Youn KH, Hur MS, Kim JS, Hu KS, Kim HJ. Clinical anatomic considerations of the zygomaticus minor muscle based on the morphology and insertion pattern. Dermatol Surg. 2014;40(8): 858–63.

28. Choi YJ, Kim JS, Gil YC, Phetudom T, Kim HJ, Tansatit T, Hu KS. Anatomic considerations regarding the location and boundary of the depressor anguli oris muscle with reference to botulinum toxin injection. Plast Reconstr Surg. 2014;134(5):917–21.

29. Hu KS, Jin GC, Youn KH, Kwak HH, Koh KS, Fontaine C, Kim HJ. An anatomic study of the bifid zygomaticus major muscle. J Craniofac Surg. 2008;19(2):534–5.

30. Hu KS, Kim ST, Hur MS, Park JH, Song WC, Koh KS, Kim HJ. Topography of the masseter muscle in relation to treatment with botulinum toxin type A. Oral Surg Oral Med Oral Pathol Oral Radiol Endod. 2010;110(2):167–71.

31. Hur MS, Hu KS, Cho JY, Kwak HH, Song WC, Koh KS, Lorente M, Kim HJ. Topography and location of the depressor anguli oris muscle with a reference to the mental foramen. Surg Radiol Anat. 2008;30(5): 403–7.

32. Hur MS, Hu KS, Kwak HH, Lee KS, Kim HJ. Inferior bundle (fourth band) of the buccinators and the incisivus labii inferioris muscle. J Craniofac Surg. 2011;22(1):289–92.

33. Hur MS, Hu KS, Park JT, Youn KH, Kim HJ. New anatomical insight of the levator labii superioris alaeque nasi and the transverse part of the nasalis. Surg Radiol Anat. 2010;32(8):753–6.

34. Hur MS, Hu KS, Youn KH, Song WC, Abe S, Kim HJ. New Anatomical profile of the nasal musculature: dilator naris vestibularis, dilator naris anterior, and alar part of the nasalis. Clin Anat. 2011; 24(2):162–7.

35. Hur MS, Kim HJ, Choi BY, Hu KS, Kim HJ, Lee KS. Morphology of the mentalis muscle and its relationship with the orbicularis oris and incisivus labii inferioris muscles. J Craniofac Surg. 2013;24(2): 602–4.

36. Hur MS, Youn KH, Hu KS, Song WC, Koh KS, Fontaine C, Kim HJ. New anatomic considerations on the levator labii superioris related with the nasal ala. J Craniofac Surg. 2010;21(1):258–60.

37. Hwang WS, Hur MS, Hu KS, Song WC, Koh KS, Baik HS, Kim ST, Kim HJ, Lee KJ. Surface anatomy of the lip elevator muscles for the treatment of gummy smile using botulinum toxin. Angle Orthod. 2009; 79(1):70–7.

38. Kim HJ, Hu KS, Kang MK, Hwang K, Chung IH. Decussation patterns of the platysma in Koreans. Br J Plast Surg. 2001;54(5):400–2.

39. Kim HS, Pae C, Bae JH, Hu KS, Chang BM, Tansatit T, Kim HJ. An anatomical study of the risorius in Asians and its insertion at the modiolus. Surg Radiol Anat. 2014;37(2):147–51.

40. Lee JY, Kim JN, Kim SH, Choi HG, Hu KS, Kim HJ, Song WC, Koh KS. Anatomical verification and designation of the superficial layer of the temporalis muscle. Clin Anat. 2012;25(2):176–81.

41. Lee JY, Kim JN, Yoo JY, Hu KS, Kim HJ, Song WC, Koh KS. Topographic anatomy of the masseter muscle focusing on the tendinous digitation. Clin Anat. 2012;25(7):889–92.

42. Park JT, Youn KH, Hu KS. Kim HJ: medial muscular band of the orbicularis oculi muscle. J Craniofac Surg. 2012;23(1):195–7.

43. Park JT, Youn KH, Hur MS, Hu KS, Kim HJ, Kim HJ. Malaris muscle, the lateral muscular band of orbicularis oculi muscle. J Craniofac Surg. 2011;22(2): 659–62.

44. Shim KS, Hu KS, Kwak HH, Youn KH, Koh KS, Fontaine C, Kim HJ. An anatomy of the insertion of the zygomaticus major muscle in human focused on the muscle arrangement at the mouth corner. Plast Reconstr Surg. 2008;121(2):466–73.

45. Yang HM, Kim HJ. Anatomical study of the corrugator supercilii muscle and its clinical implication with botulinum toxin A injection. Surg Radiol Anat. 2013;35(9):817–21.

46. Youn KH, Park JT, Park DS, Koh KS, Kim HJ, Paik DJ. Morphology of the zygomaticus minor and its relationship with the orbicularis oculi muscle. J Craniofac Surg. 2012;23(2):546–8.

47. Yu SK, Lee MH, Kim HS, Park JT, Kim HJ, Kim HJ. Histomorphologic approach for the modiolus with reference to reconstructive and aesthetic surgery. J Craniofac Surg. 2013;24(4):1414–7.

Vessels of the Face and Neck

48. Jung DH, Kim HJ, Koh KS, Oh CS, Kim KS, Yoon JH, Chung IH. Arterial supply of the nasal tip in Asians. Laryngoscope. 2000;110(2):308–11.

49. Jung W, Youn KH, Won SY, Park JT, Hu KS, Kim HJ. Clinical implications of the middle temporal vein with regard to temporal fossa augmentation. Dermatol Surg. 2014;40(6):618–23.

50. Kim YS, Choi DY, Gil YC, Hu KS, Tansatit T, Kim HJ. The anatomical origin and course of the angular artery regarding its clinical implications. Dermatol Surg. 2014;40(10):1070–6.

51. Koh KS, KIM HJ, Oh CS, Chung IH. Branching patterns and symmetry of the course of the facial artery in Koreans. Int J Oral Max Surg. 2003;32(4): 414–8.

52. Kwak HH, Hu KS, Youn KH, Jin KH, Shim KS, Fontaine C, Kim HJ. Topographic relationship between the muscle bands of the zygomaticus major muscle and the facial artery. Surg Radiol Anat. 2006;28(5):477–80.

53. Kwak HH, Jo JB, Hu KS, Oh CS, Koh KS, Chung IH, Kim HJ. Topography of the third portion of the maxillary artery via the transantral approach in Asians. J Craniofac Surg. 2010;21(4):1284–9.

54. Lee HJ, Kang IW, Won SY, Lee JG, Hu KS, Tansatit T, Kim HJ. Description of a novel anatomical venous structure in the nasoglabellar area. J Craniofac Surg. 2014;25(2):633–5.

55. Lee JG, Yang HM, Choi YJ, Favero V, Kim YS, Hu KS, Kim HJ. Facial arterial depth and layered relationship with facial musculatures. Plast Reconstr Surg. 2015;135:437–44.

56. Lee JG, Yang HM, Hu KS, Lee YI, Lee HJ, Choi YJ, Kim HJ. Frontal branch of the superficial temporal artery: anatomical study and clinical implications regarding injectable treatments. Surg Radiol Anat. 2015;37(1):61–8.

57. Lee SH, Gil YC, Choi YJ, Tansatit T, Kim HJ, Hu KS. Topographic anatomy of superior labial artery for dermal filler injection. Plast Reconstr Surg. 2015;135:445–50.

58. Lee SH, Lee M, Kim HJ. Anatomy-based image-processing analysis for the running pattern of the perioral artery for minimally invasive surgery. Br J Oral Max Surg. 2014;52(8):688–92.

59. Lee SH, Lee HJ, Kim YS, Kim HJ, Hu KS. What's difference between the inferior labial artery and horizontal labiomental artery? Surg Radiol Anat. 2015; 37(8):947–53.

60. Lee YI, Yang HM, Pyeon HJ, Lee HK, Kim HJ. Anatomical and histological study of the arterial distribution in the columellar area, and the clinical implications. Surg Radiol Anat. 2014;36(7):669–74.

61. Park KH, Kim YK, Woo SJ, Kang SW, Lee WK, Choi KS, Kwak HW, Yoon IH, Huh K, Kim JW. Iatrogenic occlusion of the ophthalmic artery after cosmetic facial filler injections: a national survey by the Korean Retina Society. JAMA Ophthalmol. 2014;132(6):714–23.

62. Yang HM, Lee JG, Hu KS, Gil YC, Choi YJ, Lee HK, Kim HJ. New anatomical insights of the course and branching patterns of the facial artery: clinical implications regarding injectable treatments to the nasolabial fold and nasojugal groove. Plast Reconstr Surg. 2014;133(5):1077–82.

63. Yang HM, Lee YI, Lee JG, Choi YJ, Lee HJ, Lee SH, Hu KS, Kim HJ. Topography of superficial arteries on the face. J Phys Anthropol. 2013;26:131–40.

64. Yang HM, Jung W, Won SY, Youn KH, Hu KS, Kim HJ. Anatomical study of medial zygomaticotemporal vein and its clinical implication regarding the injectable treatments. Surg Radiol Anat. 2014;37(2):175–80.

Peripheral Nerves of the Face and Neck

65. Hu KS, Kwak HH, Song WC, Kang HJ, Kim HC, Fontaine C, Kim HJ. Branching patterns of the infraorbital nerve and topography within the infraorbital space. J Craniofac Surg. 2006;17(6):1111–5.

66. Hu KS, Kwak J, Koh KS, Abe S, Fontaine C, Kim HJ. Topographic distribution area of the infraorbital nerve. Surg Radiol Anat. 2007;29(5):383–8.

67. Hu KS, Yun HS, Hur MS, Kwon HJ, Abe S, Kim HJ. Branching patterns and intraosseous course of the mental nerve. J Oral Maxillofac Surg. 2007;65(11): 2288–94.

68. Kim DH, Hong HS, Won SY, Kim HJ, Hu KS, Choi JH, Kim HJ. Intramuscular nerve distribution of the masseter muscle for botulinum toxin injection. J Craniofac Surg. 2010;21(2):588–91.

69. Kim HJ, Koh KS, Oh CS, Hu KS, Kang JW, Chung IH. Emerging patterns of the cervical cutaneous nerves in Asians. Int J Oral Max Surg. 2002;31(1): 53–6.

70. Kwak HH, Ko SJ, Jung HS, Park HD, Chung IH, Kim HJ. Topographic anatomy of the deep temporal nerves, with references to the superior head of lateral pterygoid. Surg Radiol Anat. 2003;25(5–6):393–9.

71. Kwak HH, Park HD, Youn KH, Hu KS, Koh KS, Han SH, Kim HJ. Branching patterns of the facial nerve and its communication with the auriculotemporal nerve. Surg Radiol Anat. 2004;26(6):494–500.

72. Lee HJ, Choi KS, Won SY, Prawit A, Hu KS, Kim ST, Tanvaa T, Kim HJ. Topographic relationship between the supratrochlear nerve and corrugator supercilii muscle for the botulinum toxin injections in chronic migraine. Toxins (Basel). 2015;7:2629–38.

73. Won SY, Kim DH, Yang HM, Park JT, Kwak HH, Hu KS, Kim HJ. Clinical and anatomical approach using Sihler's staining technique (whole mount nerve stain). Anat Cell Biol. 2011;44(1):1–7.

74. Won SY, Yang HM, Woo HS, Chang KY, Youn KH, Kim HJ, Hu KS. Neuroanastomosis and the innervation territory of the mental nerve. Clin Anat. 2014;27(4):598–602.

75. Yang HM, Won SY, Kim HJ, Hu KS. Sihler staining study of anastomosis between the facial and trigeminal nerves in the ocular area and its clinical implications. Muscle Nerve. 2013;48(4):545–50.

76. Yang HM, Won SY, Kim HJ, Hu KS. Sihler's staining study of the infraorbital nerve and its clinical complication. J Craniofac Surg. 2014;25(6):2209–13.

77. Yang HM, Won SY, Lee JG, Han SH, Kim HJ, Hu KS. Sihler-stain study of buccal nerve distribution and its clinical implications. Oral Surg Oral Med O. 2012;113(3):334–9.

Clinical Anatomy for Botulinum Toxin Injection

2

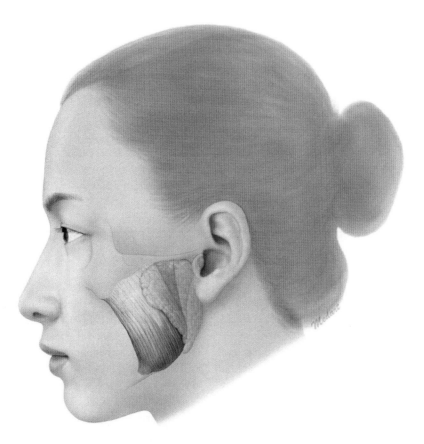

Kyle K. Seo, MD, PhD & Hee-Jin Kim, DDS, PhD (Illustrated by Kwan-Hyun Youn)

© Springer Science+Business Media Singapore 2016
H.-J. Kim et al., *Clinical Anatomy of the Face for Filler and Botulinum Toxin Injection*,
DOI 10.1007/978-981-10-0240-3_2

2.1   Introduction

2.1.1   Effective Versus Ineffective Indications of Botulinum Toxin for Wrinkle Treatment

A wrinkle, or rhytide, is categorized into dynamic and static conditions. Static wrinkles can be further divided into either fine lines or furrows/deep furrows. Dynamic wrinkles can be seen at the glabellar region when frowning or around the periorbital regions when smiling. Glabellar furrows and nasolabial folds are representative cases of deep furrows. The process of the wrinkle formation begins from dynamic wrinkles, and then the dynamic wrinkles become fixed as fine lines. With age, fine lines transform into deep furrows accompanied by a gradual loss of the underlying soft tissues.

Although botulinum toxin is often believed to be the mainstay of wrinkle treatment by general people, it cannot be applied to the treatment for all wrinkles. Main indications of botulinum toxin for wrinkle treatment are dynamic wrinkles such as forehead lines, glabellar frown lines, periorbital wrinkles, wrinkles on dorsum of the nose, fine lines around the lips, and the platysmal bands by paralyzing the underlying facial mimetic muscles. However, it is ineffective in treating furrows. Therefore, filler injections should be recommended for the treatment of furrows, including nasolabial folds, the marionette lines, and glabellar frown lines.

Some static wrinkles, such as horizontal necklines and bracelet lines, are not amenable to treatment by botulinum toxin because they are innate lines since birth. On the other hand, fine lines, which result from habitual contraction of the underlying facial mimetic muscles, can be improved with botulinum toxin injection to some extent. The representative areas where the toxin treatment can bring about improvement of fine lines include forehead, glabella, and lateral canthal area. The mechanism of botulinum toxin for improving fine lines can be hypothesized in many different ways. Firstly, it can weaken the muscle tone of underlying facial muscles attached directly to the skin. As a result, the fine lines in repose seem to improve. Secondly, the paralysis of the facial mimetic muscles attached to dermis leads to lymphatic insufficiency, and subsequent dermal edema in the skin may happen. The consequence can improve fine wrinkles and facial pores.

Botulinum toxin is ineffective in some types of dynamic wrinkles. The representative examples are transverse infraorbital wrinkles and zygomatic wrinkles which are caused by the mouth corner elevators while smiling. The botulinum toxin injection should be also avoided in the area of cheek and nasolabial folds where dynamic wrinkles are deepened during facial expression. If the botulinum toxin is injected onto these mouth corner elevators such as zygomaticus major muscle, awkward and asymmetrical smile may occur. This kind of dynamic wrinkles could be improved only by multiple intradermal injections of hyaluronic acid filler (Fig 2.1).

2.1.2   Botulinum Rebalancing

The repetitive movement of facial muscle is one of the factors contributing to the facial wrinkles. Contrary to the skeletal muscles which have muscular fascia, the facial expression muscles are not separated by fascia. Moreover, muscle fibers are directly attached to the dermis; each fiber is intermingled with complexity

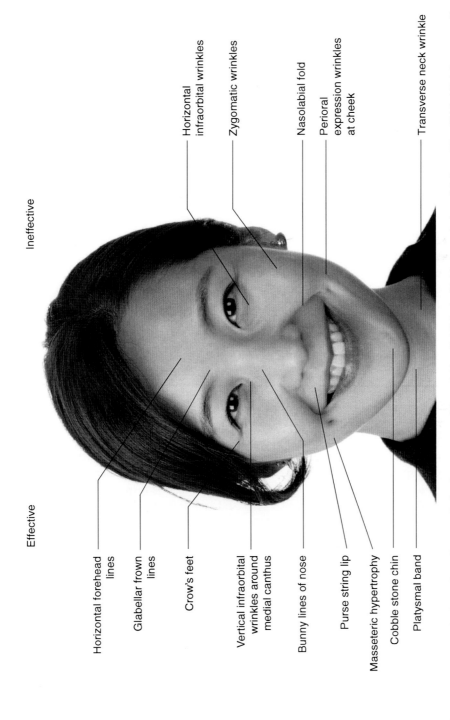

Ineffective

Horizontal
infraorbital wrinkles

Zygomatic wrinkles

Nasolabial fold

Perioral
expression wrinkles
at cheek

Transverse neck wrinkle

Effective

Horizontal forehead
lines

Glabellar frown
lines

Crow's feet

Vertical infraorbital
wrinkles around
medial canthus

Bunny lines of nose

Purse string lip

Masseteric hypertrophy

Cobble stone chin

Platysmal band

Fig. 2.1   Effective indications of botulinum toxin for the treatment of the wrinkles (Published with kind permission of © Saran Kim 2016. All rights reserved)

and continues to the SMAS (superficial musculoaponeurotic system). Thus, facial expression muscles maintain the balance of action between muscles bilaterally, upwardly, and downwardly. In patients with cardiovascular stroke, when one side of facial muscles is paralyzed, nonparalyzed muscles of the opposite site move more actively, and this results in characteristic distortion to the patients. Likewise, several delicate changes to facial expression caused by the imbalance between the facial muscles can happen from botulinum toxin. The opposite side muscles move more actively than the paralyzed side by botulinum toxin. This phenomenon could be called "botulinum rebalancing" (Fig 2.2).

The facial expression muscles are categorized into two groups: the elevators and depressors (Table 2.1). While the frontalis is the only elevator of the eyebrow, the orbicularis oculi m., corrugator supercilii m., depressor supercilii m., and procerus m. are the depressors of the eyebrow. The perioral muscles are composed of five elevators and three depressors. The perioral elevators are zygomaticus major m. (ZMj), zygomaticus minor m. (Zmi), levator labii superioris alaeque nasi m. (LLSAN), levator labii superioris m. (LLS), and levator anguli oris m. (LAO). The perioral depressors are depressor labii inferioris m. (DLI), depressor anguli oris m. (DAO), and platysma muscle.

The botulinum toxin can be effectively applied for elevating the eyebrow, mouth corner, and jowl by leveraging effect of "botulinum rebalancing." The paralysis of the depressors by botulinum toxin could lead to an elevation of the eyebrow, mouth corner, and jowl by hyperactivation of elevators. This is the mechanism of "botulinum rebalancing." The elevation of the eyebrow by weakening the depressor muscles of the eyebrow such as orbicularis oculi m., corrugator supercilii m., and procerus m. is the representative case of "botulinum rebalancing" (Fig 2.3). The elevation of the mouth corner is also performed by weakening the depressors of mouth corner. The botulinum toxin injection on the platysmal band in charge of depressing the jowl may also improve the sagging jowl to some extent.

On the other hand, the unwanted side effect of the botulinum rebalancing includes new wrinkle formation near the injected area. For example, the toxin injection only on the lateral canthal area makes the wrinkles below the medial canthal area more pronounced. The bunny lines can be exaggerated after toxin injection on the glabella area. The samurai eyebrow is another example of adverse effect of "botulinum rebalancing" when the toxin is not injected laterally to midpupillary line in case with treatment for the horizontal forehead lines.

2.2   Botulinum Wrinkle Treatment

2.2.1   Crow's Feet (Lateral Canthal Rhytides)

2.2.1.1 Target Muscle and Anatomy

The orbicularis oculi refers to the muscle around the eyes and is responsible for closing the eyelid and protecting the eyeballs. The orbicularis oculi m. (OOc) is divided into the orbital portion and the palpebral portion according to its

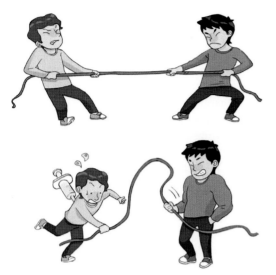

Table 2.1 Elevator and depressor muscle groups of the face

	Elevators	Depressors
Eyebrow	Frontalis	Orbicularis oculi Corrugator supercilii Depressor supercilii Procerus
Lip/jaw line	Levator labii superioris alaeque nasi (LLSAN) Levator labii superioris (LLS) Zygomaticus minor Levator anguli oris (LAO) Zygomaticus major	Depressor labii inferioris (DLI), Depressor anguli oris (DAO), Platysma

Fig. 2.2 Schematic illustration for the concept of the botulinum rebalancing (Published with kind permission of © Kwan-Hyun Youn 2016. All rights reserved)

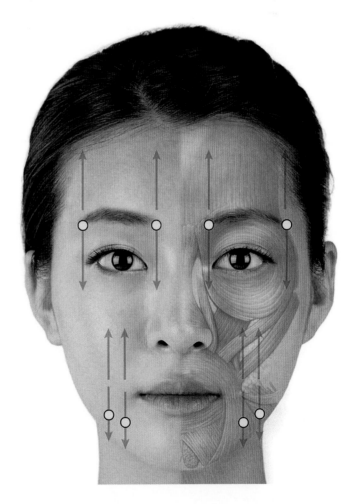

Fig. 2.3 Botulinum rebalancing O: injection points of botulinum toxin (Published with kind permission of © Kwan-Hyun Youn 2016. All rights reserved)

position. The palpebral portion is subdivided into preseptal and pretarsal portions (Fig. 2.4). The orbital portion originates from both supra-orbital and infraorbital margins and reaches the medial/lateral canthal tendon, the skin, fibers of the frontalis m., the procerus m., and the cor-rugator supercilii m. In Asians, the length from the lateral canthus to the lateral edge of the OOc was 3.1 cm on average. The lateral muscular band and the medial muscular band of the OOc were observed as 54 % and 64 %, respectively (Fig. 2.5).

Muscle fibers of the orbital portion firmly close the eyelids, pull down the eyebrows, and produce crow's feet around the outer corners of the eyes when smiling. Muscle fibers of the palpebral portion are composed of preseptal and pretarsal parts. These parts are located in the superficial layer of both the orbital septum and the tarsal plate. The palpebral portion acts involuntarily, closing the eyelids when blinking and producing vertical wrinkles in the medial canthus.

The complexly arranged fibers produce differ-ent wrinkles at each part as the OOc surrounds the circumference of the orbit. The wrinkles form horizontally at the corner of the eyes where the OOc muscle fiber runs vertically, form a 30–60° at the margin lateral to the lower eye, and form vertically at the upper eyelids where it runs hori-zontally (Fig. 2.6).

2.2.1.2 Injection Points and Methods (Fig. 2.7)

The injection landmark for crow's feet is 1.5–2 cm lateral to the lateral canthus. First, 2 U is injected at this point. 2 U is injected 0.5 cm medial and 1 cm superior to the landmark; 2 U is injected 1 cm medial and 2 cm superior to the landmark; and 1 U is injected 0.5 cm medial and 1 cm inferior to the landmark. The sum is 6–8 U, which is a satisfactory dose for each side. There is no reason to inject more than 3 cm lateral to the lateral canthus because the average length from the lateral canthus to the lateral edge of the OOc is 3.1 cm in Asians.

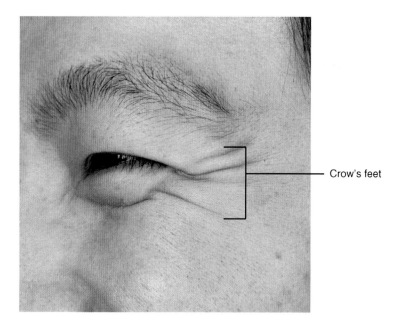

— Crow's feet

Fig. 2.4 Crow's feet and its relationships with surrounding facial muscles

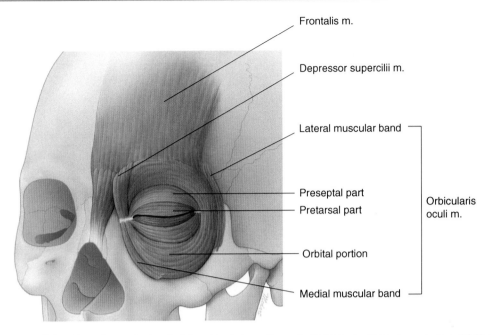

Fig. 2.5 Medial and lateral muscular band of the orbicularis oculi muscle (Published with kind permission of © Kwan-Hyun Youn 2016. All rights reserved)

Fig. 2.6 Crow's feet and its underlying muscle (Published with kind permission of © Kwan-Hyun Youn 2016. All rights reserved)

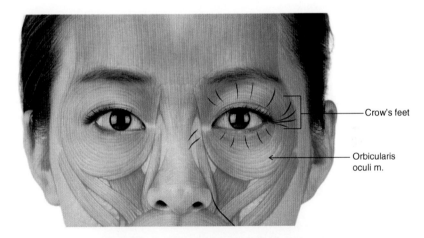

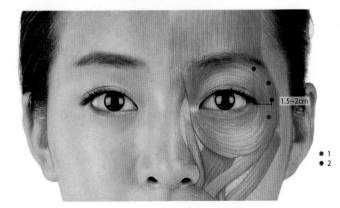

Fig. 2.7 Injection points of botulinum toxin for crow's feet (Published with kind permission of © Kwan-Hyun Youn 2016. All rights reserved)

Widening of the Eye Opening

BTA injection for widening of eye opening can remove the pretarsal bulge and slightly lower the inferior ciliary margin to widen the palpebral aperture. The procedure of widening the eye opening by injecting toxin into the lower eyelid is reported by Flynn et al. Injecting 2 U botulinum toxin into the point just below the eyelash at the midpupillary line can make the eye opening wider by 0.5 mm at resting state and by 1.3 mm during smiling, respectively. With a combined procedure of the periorbital botulinum wrinkle treatment, the eye opening can be widened up to 1.8 mm and 2.9 mm, respectively.

From the view point of Caucasians, this treatment may help Asians' smaller eyes to become bigger. Actually, this treatment is appealing to some Southeast Asians who regard almond-shaped eyes as a beautiful hallmark. However, it is important not to apply this treatment to East Asians, who consider pretarsal bulge one of the important hallmarks of female beauty. The pretarsal muscular bulge is usually exaggerated during smiling by the action of orbicularis oculi muscle. Therefore, it is called as "charming roll" in East Asians because the people with pretarsal muscular bulge in repose look soft

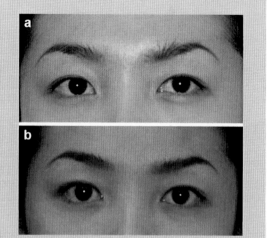

Fig. 2.8 Before (**a**) and 1 week after (**b**) injection of botulinum toxin for widening of eye opening (Published with kind permission of © Kyle K Seo 2016. All rights reserved)

and friendly. Another reason for explaining the popularity of "charming roll" in East Asians is that the "charming roll" brings the optical illusion of a "big eye" like double eye surgery in Asians with inherently smaller eyes. Therefore, physicians even enhance "charming roll" by the injection of filler in Asians. In such a context, BTA injection for widening of the eye opening should be avoided in East Asians (Fig. 2.8).

2.2.2 Infraorbital Wrinkles

Infraorbital wrinkles are divided into infraorbital horizontal wrinkles, the medial epicanthal fold, and the lateral epicanthal fold. Infraorbital horizontal wrinkles are produced by the zygomaticus major m., which pulls up the zygomatic soft tissue when smiling. The zygomaticus major m. lifts the mouth corner. As long as this muscle contracts, toxin is not useful. But, the "medial epicanthal fold," or the horizontal wrinkle is

formed inferior to the medial canthus by the orbicularis oculi m. The botulinum toxin is an appropriate treatment for these dynamic wrinkles (Fig. 2.9). Injecting into the eye rim area may cause "botulinum rebalancing" in order to eliminate crow's feet around the eyes since muscles related to facial expressions are connected to each other. Due to the botulinum-rebalancing phenomenon, hypercontraction of the inferior orbicularis oculi m. may lead to horizontal lines below the eyes, especially the area inferior to the

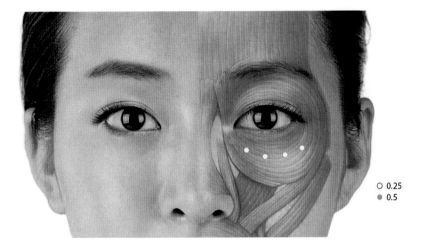

Fig. 2.9 Injection points of the botulinum toxin for infraorbital wrinkles (Published with kind permission of © Kwan-Hyun Youn 2016. All rights reserved)

○ 0.25
● 0.5

medial canthus area. For this reason, 1–2 U is injected vertically into the muscle fibers on the border between preseptal part of palpebral portion and orbital portion, ranging from the inferior medial canthus to the lateral canthus, to avoid the botulinum-rebalancing phenomenon when injecting into the lateral canthal rhytides (Fig. 2.9).

2.2.3 Horizontal Forehead Lines

2.2.3.1 Target Muscle and Anatomy
(Fig. 2.10)

The frontalis m., which forms horizontal forehead lines, originates from the galea aponeurotica near the coronal suture. These muscle fibers intertwine with fibers of the superciliary arch, the procerus, the corrugator supercilii, and the orbicularis oculi muscle. The frontalis runs inferomedially. The upper medial part of the frontalis is attached to the aponeurosis more inferiorly than the lateral part. For this reason, the upper medial part of the forehead shows a V-shape about 3.5 cm above the superciliary arch. Thus, a little amount of the toxin is necessary, or no injection is needed for this V-shaped part.

2.2.3.2 Injection Points and Method
(Fig. 2.11)

The most commonly used dosage in this muscle is 6 U; however, a half dose should be injected when a blepharoptosis or an eyebrow ptosis exists.

2.2.4 Glabellar Frown Lines

2.2.4.1 Target Muscle and Anatomy
(Fig. 2.12)

Glabellar lines are created by three muscles: the frontalis, the procerus, and the corrugator supercilii muscle (CSM). Superomedial fibers of the orbicularis oculi, also known as the depressor supercilii, are intertwined with the frontalis and the procerus. The CSM originates from the superomedial aspect of the orbital rim and passes superolaterally at 30° to attach to the dermis at the middle of the eyebrow. The CSM draws the eyebrow inferiorly and medially, producing vertical wrinkles on the forehead as when frowning. The CSM is found beneath the frontalis because its origin is the frontal bone.

The procerus m. originates from the nasal bone and the upper part of the lateral nasal cartilage. Its fibers run vertically by merging with fibers of the frontalis with some of them attaching to the skin over the radix and glabella area. The depressor supercilii m., the medial part of the orbicularis oculi m., draws the eyebrows down. If this muscle is injected with botulinum toxin, the eyebrows can be lifted upward. The muscles of the glabella are not separated but actually intertwined with each other, and the toxin diffuses to the underlying muscle. Thus, injecting into the CSM can paralyze other neighboring muscles in the glabellar area.

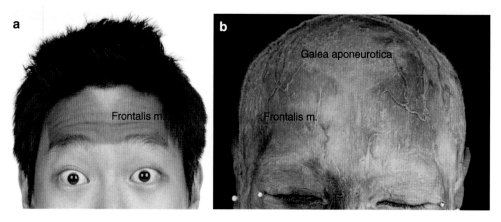

Fig. 2.10 Frontalis muscle on the forehead (**a, b**) (Published with kind permission of © Hee-Jin Kim and Kwan-Hyun Youn 2016. All rights reserved)

Fig. 2.11 Injection points of the botulinum toxin horizontal forehead lines (Published with kind permission of © Kwan-Hyun Youn 2016. All rights reserved)

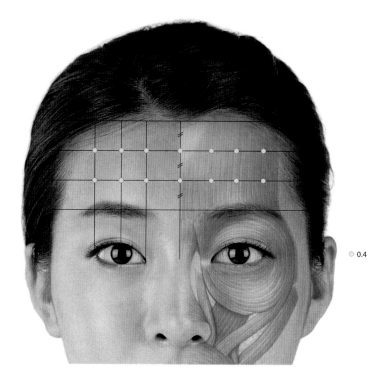

Tip: Screening High-Risk Patients of Botulinum Forehead Wrinkle Removal

1. Patients in their late 40s or over
2. Patients with blepharoptosis
3. Patients raising their eyebrow with frontalis m.

Patients whose forehead wrinkles intensify when opening their eyes. Patients having difficulty in opening their eyes when upper area of the eyebrow is pressed

4. Patients with thick and swollen eyelids
5. Men with single eyelids

Clinical Anatomy of the Corrugator Supercilii M. in Asians

The corrugator supercilii m. of Koreans arises from 16 mm above the horizontal intercanthal plane (HL) and 4–14 mm from the midline on average and interlaces into the frontalis m. and the dermis 30 mm above the HL and 16–35 mm from the midline. The maximum vertical length of corrugator supercilii m. of Koreans is slightly shorter compared to that of Caucasians, the length of each being 15 mm and 21 mm, respectively. The corrugator supercilii m. morphologically consists of two clearly distinct bellies, the oblique belly (OB) and the transverse belly (TB). The OB arises from the upper side, while the TB arises from the superolateral aspect, running horizontally. There are two types of OB, the narrow vertical type and the broad triangular type (Fig. 2.12). The oblique belly of the narrow vertical type extended superiorly and had a narrow rectangular shape. This muscle belly reached the frontalis m. at the superomedial orbital part, near the glabella area and within the medial one-third of the transverse belly (63 %). The broad triangular type was observed as a triangular-shaped belly covering the medial half of the transverse belly. The oblique belly of the broad triangular type covered the medial half of the transverse belly (37 %) (Fig. 2.13). It is presumed that people whose OB is more developed show more muscle contraction of the eyebrow above the midpupillary line.

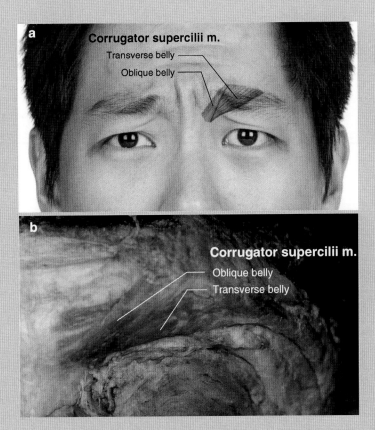

Fig. 2.12 Glabellar frown lines and its corresponding corrugator supercilii muscle (**a, b**) (Published with kind permission of © Hee-Jin Kim and Kwan-Hyun Youn 2016. All rights reserved)

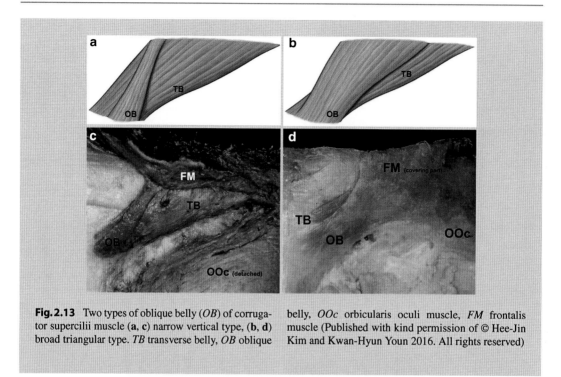

Fig. 2.13 Two types of oblique belly (*OB*) of corrugator supercilii muscle (**a, c**) narrow vertical type, (**b, d**) broad triangular type. *TB* transverse belly, *OB* oblique belly, *OOc* orbicularis oculi muscle, *FM* frontalis muscle (Published with kind permission of © Hee-Jin Kim and Kwan-Hyun Youn 2016. All rights reserved)

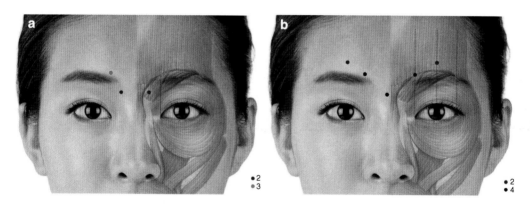

Fig. 2.14 Injection points of botulinum toxin for glabellar frown lines (**a**) standard form for Asian, (**b**) severe form for Caucasian (Published with kind permission of © Kwan-Hyun Youn 2016. All rights reserved)

2.2.4.2 Injection Points and Methods

It is recommended that an injection be made into the CSM after the needle tip comes into contact with the frontal bone and is slightly withdrawn since the CSM is located deep inside. 3 U (4 U for male) is injected around the upper border of the medial orbital rim just above the medial canthus, the insertion area for the CSM. 2 U is injected into the midpoint between the insertion area of the depressor supercilii and the nasion (intercanthal midpoint) in order to treat the procerus and the depressor supercilii m. on each side (standard form for Asian (Fig. 2.14a)).

In Asians, the narrow vertical type of the oblique belly (OB) of the CSM is found in 63 % more frequently than 37 % of the broad triangular type. Moreover, the OB length is shorter than that of Caucasians. Therefore, injection of toxin only into the medial part of CSM as shown in a standard form for Asians would be sufficient in Asians compared to the standard form for Caucasians which includes injection points just above the brow in the midpupillary line. However, if patients show active movement above the eyebrows in the midpupillary line when making glabellar expression lines, 1 U per side should be injected intradermally into the same injection points above the brow in the midpupillary line, as in Caucasians (Fig. 2.14b).

Palpebral Ptosis (Fig. 2.15)

The thing to be most cautious when treating glabellar frown line is blepharoptosis. This symptom occurs as the toxin injected into the corrugator supercilii m. spreads to the levator palpebrae superioris m. through the orbital septum, causing the levator palpebrae superioris m. to partially paralyze. In order to prevent blepharoptosis, the direction of the injection needle is crucial: it should point upward and lateral along the corrugator supercilii m.

However, if blepharoptosis does occur, it is recommended that α-symphathomimetic eyedrops are used 3–4 times a day as symptomatic treatment. The Müller m., or tarsal m., which pulls up the eyelid, is situated between the levator palpebrae superioris m. and palpebral conjunctiva and assists the levator palpebrae superioris m. Sympathetic nerves are distributed in the Müller m. When 0.5 % Iopidine eyedrops, which are α-symphathomimetics, are applied, the apraclonidine that is absorbed through the mucous membrane of the eyes immediately affects the Müller m., and the upper eyelids can be lifted 1–2 mm.

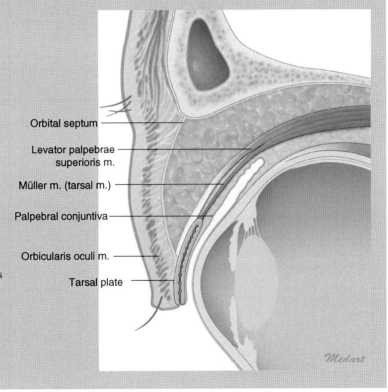

Fig. 2.15 Sagittal section of the upper eyelid and eyeball showing the relationship between levator palpebrae superioris muscle and Müller muscle (or tarsal muscle) related with ptosis after botulinum toxin injection (Published with kind permission of © Kwan-Hyun Youn 2016. All rights reserved)

Orbital septum

Levator palpebrae superioris m.

Müller m. (tarsal m.)

Palpebral conjuntiva

Orbicularis oculi m.

Tarsal plate

Tip: Ways for the Absolute Prevention of Palpebral Ptosis

To prevent blepharoptosis, the doctor should pay close attention to factors such as the dose of botulinum toxin, concentration, direction of the needle, location and velocity of the injection, position of the doctor and patient, and position of the hand.

1. Location of the injection

   The location of the injection is of utmost importance in preventing blepharoptosis and should be as superior as possible from the boundary of the orbital rim . The place that the corrugator supercilii m. arises is located right above the upper inner boundary of the orbital rim. It is possible that the contents of the injection might spread into the orbital rim if directly injected where the corrugator supercilii m. arises, so the needle should be injected 1 cm superior to the upper inner boundary of the orbital rim.

   Botulinum toxin spreads about 1 cm, so it is okay to inject a bit above the location where the corrugator supercilii m. arises. Many clinicians inject based on the eyebrows, as the eyebrows are usually situated along the upper inner boundary of the orbital rim. However, if the place of injection is chosen based on the eyebrows, there is a higher possibility of blepharoptosis for patients over 50s with eyebrow ptosis, as the injection may have been lower than the boundary of the orbital rim. Therefore, check the boundary of the orbital rim with the fingertip first and then perform the injection perpendicular to the inner ocular angle instead of the eyebrow for patients with eyebrow ptosis.

2. Dose

   If a big dose is injected, it may spread downward. Therefore, the concentration should be maintained at 4 U/0.1 mL, and a single injection should not exceed 4 U.

3. Direction of the needle

   The direction of the needle should point toward the upper lateral side so that the botulinum toxin does not spread inside the orbital rim at a 30° angle from both the eyebrow horizon and the surface of the skin.

4. Velocity

   Inject slowly in order to prevent the toxin from flowing down to the eyelids due to pressure while injecting, pressing down and blocking firmly along the inner boundary of the orbital rim with the hand not holding the syringe. The needle should be pointing upward.

5. Position of the injector

   The doctor should stand on the left or right side of the patient while the patient is sitting, facing the patient when performing the injection. The direction of the needle should point to the upper lateral side so that the injection does not go toward the eyes. Therefore, when performing injection on the left side muscle, stand on the right side of the patient, and when performing injection on the right side muscle, stand on the left side of the patient.

6. Position of Patients

   In the beginning years, patients were advised to not lie down for 3–4 h after the glabellar line removal procedure had taken place. This was first advocated by Michael Jackson's doctor Arnold Klein in 1999. These days, however, there are no specific restrictions concerning the position of patients, as some claim that lying down can prevent the toxin from spreading downward.

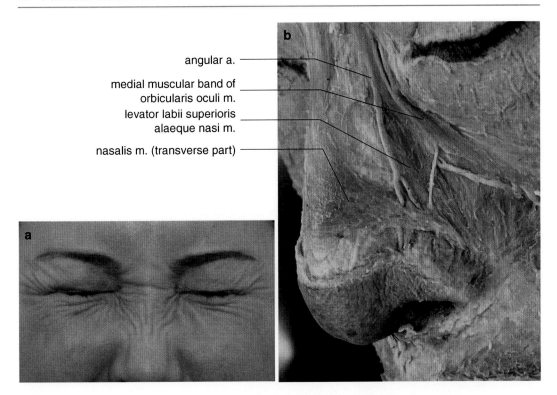

angular a.

medial muscular band of
orbicularis oculi m.

levator labii superioris
alaeque nasi m.

nasalis m. (transverse part)

Fig. 2.16 Bunny lines nasalis (**a**) and levator labii superioris alaeque nasi muscle producing bunny lines (**b**) (Published with kind permission of © Kyle K Seo and Hee-Jin Kim 2016. All rights reserved)

2.2.5 **Bunny Lines** (Fig. 2.16)

2.2.5.1 **Target Muscle and Anatomy**
A bunny line is a horizontal wrinkle that appears on both lateral and dorsal aspects of the nose when smiling and frowning. The nasalis m. produces horizontal lines on the middle of nasal dorsum; however, the levator labii superioris alaeque nasi m. (LLSAN) and the additional medial muscular band of the orbicularis oculi muscle produce bunny lines, which form on the sides of the nose. In Asians, this muscular band was observed in 66 %.

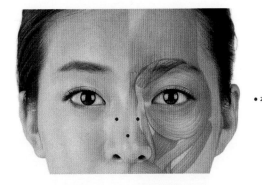

Fig. 2.17 Injection points of botulinum toxin for bunny lines (Published with kind permission of © Kwan-Hyun Youn 2016. All rights reserved)

2.2.5.2 **Injection Points and Methods**
2 U is injected into three points: the nasal dorsum and both the lateral sides (Fig. 2.17). In the strict sense, bunny lines cannot be completely removed because the muscle fibers of the LLSAN cannot be entirely paralyzed.

2.2.6   Plunged Tip of the Nose

2.2.6.1 Target Muscle and Anatomy
(Fig. 2.18a)

People with well-developed nasalis m. or depressor septi nasi, which draws the tip of the nose downward, usually present a drooping nasal tip. A toxin injection could be useful in weakening these muscles by allowing them to lift the nasal tip a little. If the patients present a drooping nasal tip when smiling, it is effective to inject into the LLSAN as well as the depressor septi.

The depressor septi located deeply on the upper lip arises from the incisive fossa of the maxilla and inserts into the movable part of nasal septum (Fig. 2.18b). The depressor septi drops the tip of the nose when contracted; therefore, the tip of the nose may be flattened, and the nostril may appear larger when smiling.

2.2.6.2 Injection Points and Methods

4 U is injected into the subnasale inferior to the columella and the ala of the nose at both sides with a total of 12 U doses. Additionally, 2 U is

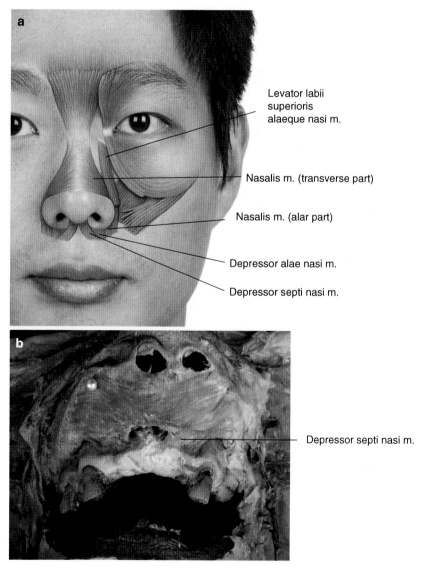

Levator labii superioris alaeque nasi m.

Nasalis m. (transverse part)

Nasalis m. (alar part)

Depressor alae nasi m.

Depressor septi nasi m.

Depressor septi nasi m.

Fig. 2.18 Muscles of the nose (**a**) and depressor septi nasi muscle on the dissected specimen (**b**) (Published with kind permission of © Hee-Jin Kim and Kwan-Hyun Youn 2016. All rights reserved)

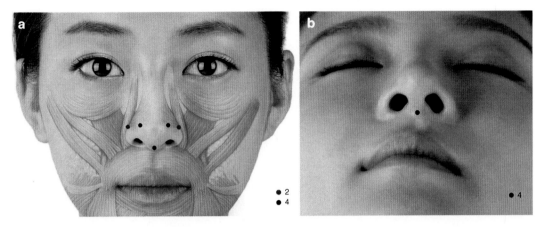

Fig. 2.19 Injection points of botulinum toxin for plunged tip of the nose (**a**, **b**) (Published with kind permission of © Kwan-Hyun Youn 2016. All rights reserved)

injected into the LLSAN at each side only if the patients present a drooping nasal tip when smiling (Fig. 2.19).

2.2.7 Gummy Smile, Excessive Gingival Display

2.2.7.1 Target Muscle and Anatomy

The LLSAN, the LLS, and the Zmi determine the amount of lip elevation that occurs upon smiling. Gums are revealed upon smiling when these muscles are hyperactive. Among these, the LLSAN originates from the frontal process of the maxilla and the maxillary process of the frontal bone. It then runs down vertically and inserts into the mid-central part of the orbicularis oris, the nasal ala, and the skin tissue of the ala of the nose. It pulls the middle of the upper lip upward and pulls the nasal ala both upward and laterally. Therefore, it is involved in forming the medial most upper portion of the nasolabial fold. It also pulls the tip of the nose down, which is also known as the ptotic nose (Fig. 2.20).

The LLS originates from the orbital rim of the maxilla and inserts into the upper lip. Most muscle fibers of the medial 1/2 LLS are also attached to the ala of the nose (90%). Therefore, the LLSAN and the LLS not only pull the middle of the upper lip upward but also pull the nasal ala both upward and laterally. Among these muscles, which draw up the upper lip, the LLS is located deep inside, the LLSAN lays mediosuperiorly,

and the Zmi lies laterally. In Koreans, the mean angle between the facial midline and each muscle vector was −20° for the LLSAN, 26° for the LLS, and 56° for the Zmi. These three muscles converge lateral to the ala of the nose and are intertwined at the upper lip.

2.2.7.2 Injection Points and Methods

The principle for gummy smile treatment using toxin weakens these three lip elevator muscles. But if the LLS and the Zmi are all weakened, asymmetries or upper lip drooping may occur when smiling. It is advised to paralyze some of the LLSAN. 1–2 U is injected shallowly into the point just lateral to the upper margin of the ala (Fig. 2.21a).

On the other hand, an alternative injection technique for gummy smile can be used in severe cases. Injection can be suggested as an appropriate injection point for toxin at Yonsei point, 1 cm lateral (1 finger width) from the nasal ala at the level of the nasal base (Fig. 2.21b). Single injection of 2.0 U should be done into the muscle layer and targets the whole of LLSAN, LLS, and ZMi.

2.2.8 Nasolabial Fold

2.2.8.1 Target Muscle and Anatomy

The most common treatments for nasolabial fold correction are injectable fillers; however, a toxin injection could improve a deepened nasolabial fold when smiling or an asymmetric animation of the face.

levator labii superioris alaeque nasi m. ——
levator labii superioris m. ——
zygomaticus minor m. ——
zygomaticus major m. ——

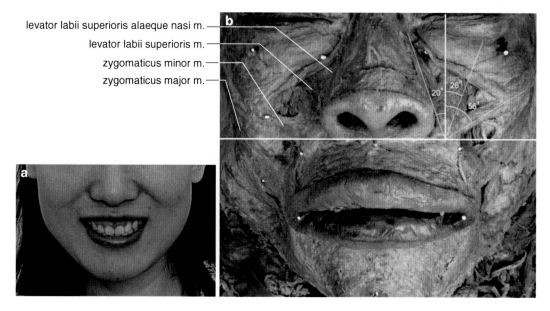

Fig. 2.20 Gummy smile (**a**). The direction of the upper lip elevator muscles to the midline (**b**) (Published with kind permission of © Kyle K Seo and Hee-Jin Kim 2016. All rights reserved)

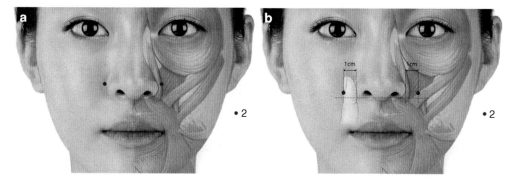

Fig. 2.21 Injection points of botulinum toxin for gummy smile. (**a**) Standard injection points for gummy smile, (**b**) alternative injection points for gummy smile (Published

with kind permission of © Kwan-Hyun Youn 2016. All rights reserved)

The object muscles at the nasolabial level are the LLSAN, the LLS, the Zmi, and the ZMj. The fibers of these muscles are attached to the skin tissue around the nasolabial fold, and the border of the nasolabial fold is formed by these muscular fibers (Fig. 2.22). The area medial to the attached line of these muscle fibers has much thinner nasolabial fat in comparison to the area superolateral to this line.

2.2.8.2 Injection Points and Methods
The principles for the treatment of the nasolabial fold are individualized approaches for the mus-

cles, such as the LLSAN, the LLS, the Zmi, and the ZMj. But, injecting only into the LLSAN is a safe way to prevent severe facial expression changes. 1–2 U is injected into the point just lateral to the upper margin of the ala (Fig. 2.23).

2.2.9 Asymmetric Smile, Facial Palsy

2.2.9.1 Target Muscle and Anatomy
Botulinum toxin injection into the Zmj is the basic treatment for an asymmetric smile and is generally injected to the more severe and

Fig. 2.22 The cutaneous insertions of upper lip elevators along nasolabial fold. Upper lip elevators (levator labii superioris alaeque nasi muscle [LLSAN], levator labii superioris muscle [LLS], zygomaticus minor muscle [Zmi], and zygomaticus major muscle [ZMj]) show the cutaneous insertion of muscle fibers along the nasolabial fold. The branches of the facial artery pass through these muscle fibers under the nasolabial fold (**a**, **b**) (Published with kind permission of © Hee-Jin Kim 2016. All rights reserved)

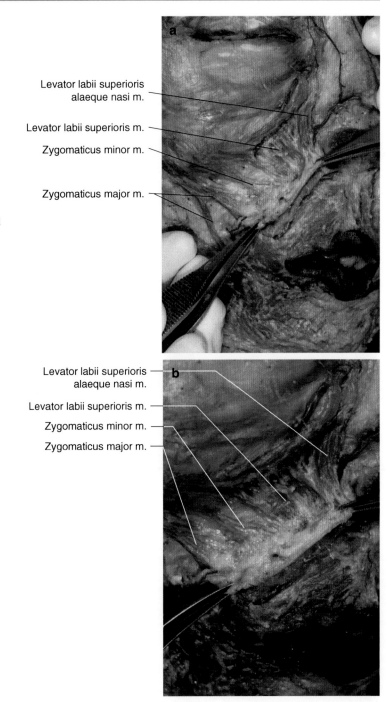

abnormal side. Injections to the normal side of the face in facial palsy patients can improve lower face symmetry when smiling and laughing.

The zygomaticus major m. originates from the facial side of the zygoma, runs both inferiorly and medially to the angle of the mouth, and contributes to the modiolus. The attachment patterns

Fig. 2.23 Injection points of botulinum toxin for nasolabial fold (Published with kind permission of © Kwan-Hyun Youn 2016. All rights reserved)

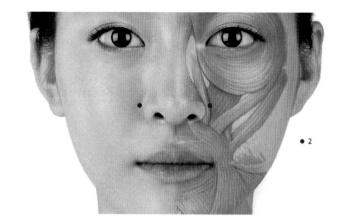

Fig. 2.24 A dissection of the modiolar region from the posterior aspect (*left side*). The deep muscle bands (*asterisk*) of the zygomaticus major (*ZMj*) muscle insertion and interlace into the deep fibers of the orbicularis oris (*OOr*) and depressor anguli oris (*DAO*) muscles. The deep muscle bands are (*asterisk*) also partially attached to the buccinator (*Buc*) muscle and its fascia (Published with kind permission of © Kwan-Hyun Youn 2016. All rights reserved)

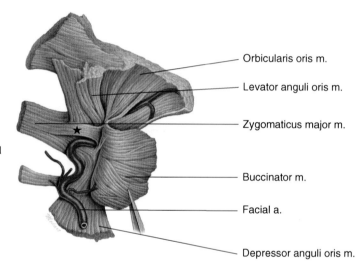

— Orbicularis oris m.

— Levator anguli oris m.

— Zygomaticus major m.

— Buccinator m.

— Facial a.

— Depressor anguli oris m.

of this muscle vary and run deeper than the levator anguli oris. The muscle fibers attached to the anterior portion of the buccinator can be observed at all times (Fig. 2.24).

2.2.9.2 Injection Points and Methods

2–4 U is deeply injected into the meeting point, located at the midline between the ala of the nose and the upper lip and at the horizontal line passing the lateral canthus, since the position of the modiolus in Koreans is placed lower than that in Caucasians (Fig. 2.25).

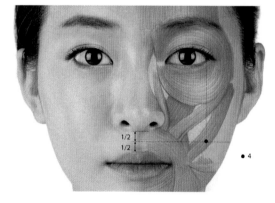

Fig. 2.25 Injection point of botulinum toxin for asymmetric smile (Published with kind permission of © Kwan-Hyun Youn 2016. All rights reserved)

2.2.10 Alar Band

2.2.10.1 Target Muscle and Anatomy

The zygomaticus minor (Zmi) originates from the zygomatic bone and inserts into the upper lip. In 28 % of Koreans, the Zmi was attached to both the upper lip and the lateral alar region. This finding of Zmi fibers being attached to the alar region suggests that this muscle is involved in the elevation of both the nasal ala and the upper lip during various facial animations. The additional insertion into the nasal ala from the Zmi forms a small protrusion (alar band) next to it as well (Fig. 2.26). In particular, the alar band appears more prominently in females with thin skin.

2.2.10.2 Injection Points and Methods

Shallow injection of 2 U into the alar band can be effective in attenuating a small protrusion by the Zmi.

2.2.11 Purse String Lip

2.2.11.1 Target Muscle and Anatomy
(Fig. 2.27)

The orbicularis oris m., the mouth's sphincter muscle, encircles the mouth. It is responsible for puckering the lips and closing the muscle. It inserts directly into facial muscular fibers and originates from the alveolar bone near the incisors of the maxilla and the mandible. It is also called the incisivus labii superioris m. or incisivus labii inferioris m.

2.2.11.2 Injection Points and Methods
(Fig. 2.28)

1 U is shallowly injected into the areas one-thirds and two-thirds between the philtrum border and the mouth angle, located 1–2 mm superior to the vermilion border, with a total of 4 U on both sides. 4 U may be injected into the inferior border of the lower lip when severe wrinkles form in that area.

2.2.12 Drooping of the Mouth Corner

2.2.12.1 Target Muscle and Anatomy

Muscles that pull the mouth corner upward and downward are balanced at the modiolus. Botulinum toxin has been used to elevate the corner of the mouth by relaxing the drooping muscle (Fig. 2.29), also called the depressor anguli oris m. (DAO). This is the so-called botulinum rebalancing.

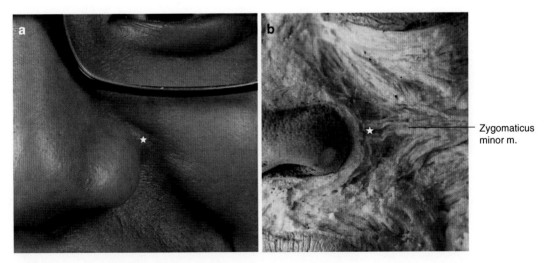

Fig. 2.26 Alar band (**a**) and its corresponding muscle fibers from zygomaticus minor inserted into the nasal ala (**b**) (Published with kind permission of © Hee-Jin Kim 2016. All rights reserved)

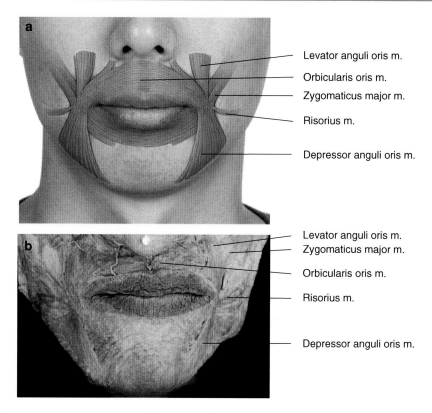

Levator anguli oris m.
Orbicularis oris m.
Zygomaticus major m.
Risorius m.

Depressor anguli oris m.

Levator anguli oris m.
Zygomaticus major m.
Orbicularis oris m.
Risorius m.

Depressor anguli oris m.

Fig. 2.27 Superficial perioral muscles (**a**, **b**) (Published with kind permission of © Hee-Jin Kim and Kwan-Hyun Youn 2016. All rights reserved)

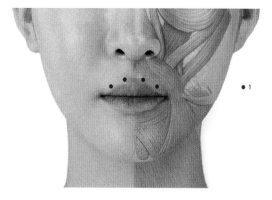

Fig. 2.28 Injection points of botulinum toxin for purse string lip (Published with kind permission of © Kwan-Hyun Youn 2016. All rights reserved)

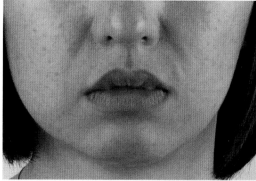

Fig. 2.29 Drooping of the mouth corner (Published with kind permission of © Hee-Jin Kim 2016. All rights reserved)

The DAO, which is triangular-shaped, arises from the oblique line of the mandible where its fibers converge with depressor labii inferioris muscle fibers. The DAO inserts into the modiolus and interlaces with the orbicularis oris and the risorius. The inferior and medial borderline in Koreans is located 1.5 cm lateral to the mandibular symphysis. The inferior width of the DAO is known to be 3.6 cm on average (Fig. 2.30).

2.2.12.2 Anatomy of Muscles Around the Mouth

The muscles that control the mouth are located on both sides located around the orbicularis oris m. with a total of 24 muscles. These muscles consist of five elevators ([LLSAN], [LLS], [Zmi], [ZMj], [LAO]), three depressors ([DAO], [DLI], [platysma m.]), two muscles laterally pulling the angle of the mouth ([risorius m.], [buccinator m.]), and the mentalis m. (Fig. 2.31). The muscles interlacing at the modiolus are divided into four layers, composed of three superficial layers and one deep layer (Table 2.2).

The traditional guideline for Caucasians suggests that the toxin be injected 1 cm lateral and 1 cm inferior to the corner of the mouth when injecting the toxin into the DAO to pull up the angle of the mouth in Caucasians. In Asians, however, injection points of the toxin are 1/3 inferior to the DAO and close to the origin of the DAO. This is because the modiolus generally lies lower in Asians than in Caucasians. When the toxin is injected at a point lateral to the DAO according to the guideline for Caucasians, the muscles attached to the modiolus, such as ZMj and the risorius m., may be influenced, resulting in unwanted changes or other difficulties related to facial animation. Therefore, it is safer and more effective to inject into the lower part of the DAO in Asians, contrary to the case in Caucasians. Facial n. branches are more compactly distributed 1/3 inferior to the DAO, the most effective area for toxin injection.

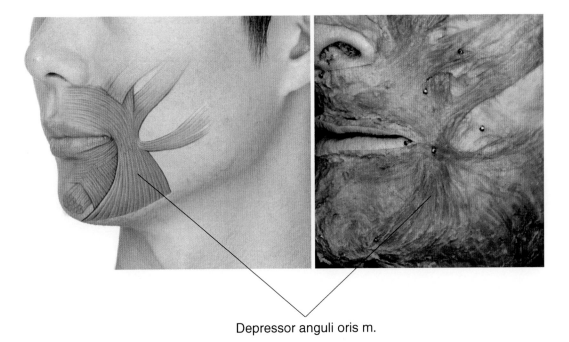

Depressor anguli oris m.

Fig. 2.30 Depressor anguli oris muscle (Published with kind permission of © Hee-Jin Kim and Kwan-Hyun Youn 2016. All rights reserved)

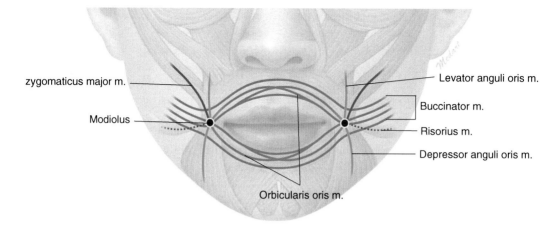

zygomaticus major m.
Modiolus
Orbicularis oris m.
Levator anguli oris m.
Buccinator m.
Risorius m.
Depressor anguli oris m.

Fig. 2.31 A schematic illustration of the muscles interlacing at the modiolus (Published with kind permission of © Kwan-Hyun Youn 2016. All rights reserved) – 지시선 다시

Table 2.2 The layers of the periorbital musculature

Superficial layer (3 separate layers)	
First layer	DAO, Risorius, OOr (superficial), ZMj (superficial)
Second layer	Platysma m., Zmi, LLSAN
Third layer	LLS, DLI, OOr (deep)
Deep layer	
Fourth layer	LAO, mentalis m., ZMj (deep), buccinators m.

DAO depressor anguli oris m., *OOr* orbicularis oris m., *ZMj* zygomaticus major m., *Zmi* zygomaticus minor m., *LLSAN* levator labii superioris alaeque nasi m., *LLS* levator labii superioris m., *DLI* depressor labii inferioris m., *LAO* levator anguli oris m.

Modiolus

The modiolus, placed laterally to the mouth corner, is derived from Latin meaning the hub of a wheel. It is a muscular structure that decussates between the orbicularis oris m. and labial tractors ending at the lateral border of the mouth corner (Fig. 2.32).

The modiolus is a dense, thick, muscular mass formed by interlacing the muscle fibers converging toward the mouth corner with the zygomaticus major, levator anguli oris, depressor anguli oris, risorius, buccinators, and orbicularis oris mm. in a vertical and a horizontal direction. The tendinous tissue nodule in the modiolus was found in 21.4 % with dense, irregular, collagenous connective tissue (Fig. 2.33). Likewise, the modiolus is a common attachment site for several muscles around the mouth. It holds an important role

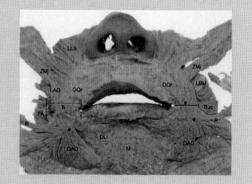

Fig. 2.32 Modiolus and converging muscles around the modiolus. *Black circle* modiolus, *yellow asterisk* cheilion, *Buc* buccinator m., *DAO* depressor anguli oris m., *DLI* depressor labii inferioris m., *FA* facial artery, *LAO* levator anguli oris m., *LBM* lateral border of the modiolus, *LLS* levator labii superioris m., *M* mentalis m., *OOr* orbicularis oris m., *R* risorius m., *ZMj* zygomaticus major m. (Published with kind permission of © Hee-Jin Kim 2016. All rights reserved)

in making facial expressions, such as sadness or happiness, and the formation of the naso-labial fold.

Contrary to the case of Caucasians, the location of the modiolus in Asians is below the intercheilion line in 58.4 % (Fig. 2.34). In

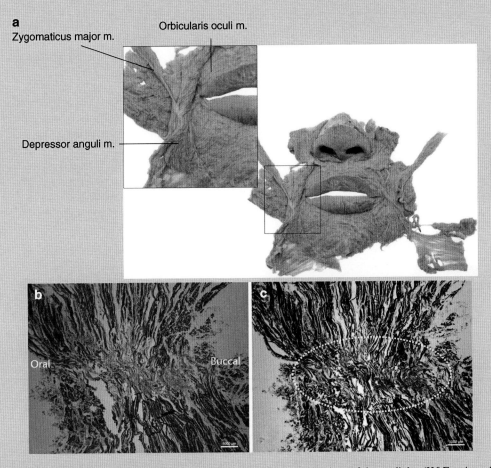

Fig. 2.33 Tendinous structure of the modiolus (**a**) and the histologic sections of the modiolus (H&E stain and Masson's trichrome stain) (**b**, **c**) (Published with kind permission of © Hee-Jin Kim 2016. All rights reserved)

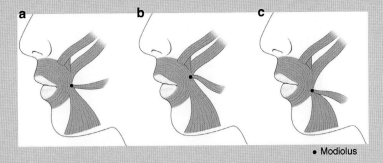

Fig. 2.34 Modiolus patterns and locations based on the level of the intercheilion horizontal line. (**a**) Modiolus located at the level of the intercheilion line, (**b**) modiolus located above the level of the intercheilion line, (**c**) modiolus located below the level of the intercheilion line (Published with kind permission of © Kwan-Hyun Youn 2016. All rights reserved)

particular, the lateral border of the modiolus is situated at a distance about 15 mm from the cheilion, 10–20 mm lateral to the mouth corner, and 10 mm inferior to the cheilion. Fibers of the ZMj are relatively longer, and the direction of the muscle fiber is more vertically located because the modiolus is placed below the intercheilion in Asians. Therefore, it is thought that the Mona Lisa smile type is more prominent in Asians.

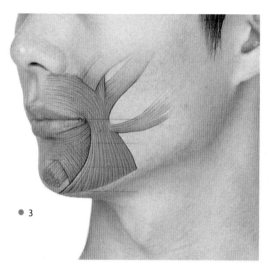

● 3

2.2.12.3 Injection Points and Methods

The injection points are 1/3 inferior to the DAO at a location coming down from a point 1 cm lateral to the mouth corner. Subdermal injections should be carried out very superficially since the DAO is the thinnest muscle. 3–4 U is the proper doses (Fig. 2.35).

2.2.13 Cobblestone Chin (Fig. 2.36)

2.2.13.1 Target Muscle and Anatomy

The mentalis m. (MT) is the only elevator for the lower lip and the chin, and it provides major vertical support for the lower lip. This muscle originates from the alveolar bone, which is inferior to the lateral incisor. The medial fibers of both MTs descend anteromedially and cross together, form-

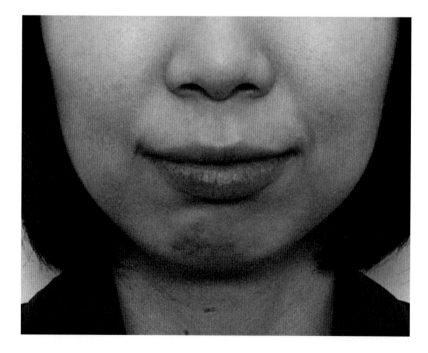

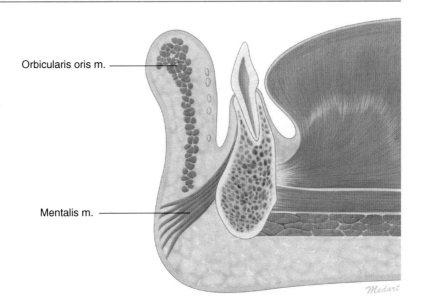

Fig. 2.37 Sagittal section of the chin showing the mentalis muscle's cutaneous insertion (Published with kind permission of © Kwan-Hyun Youn 2016. All rights reserved)

Orbicularis oris m. —

Mentalis m. —

ing a prominent dome-shaped chin (Fig. 2.37). The lateral fibers of the MT descend obliquely and cross the midline to attach to the skin on the same side. The MT contraction forms mental creases at the tip of the chin. The upper fibers of the MT run horizontally and intermingle with the inferior margin of the OOr, forming a continuous structure with the OOr. These continuous arrangements can help the MT support and raise the lip. The lateral fibers of the MT intermingle with the depressor labii inferioris muscle (Fig. 2.38).

In Asians, the average length and width of the MT is 2.0 and 1.2 cm. The MT originates from the alveolar bone 2 cm inferior to the inter-cheilion line. The origin of the MT is located 0.5–1.3 cm (average width 0.8 cm) lateral to the midline of mandible. The MT insertion is located closer to the midline rather than the origin, and the average width is approximately 0.7 cm (Fig. 2.38).

2.2.13.2 Injection Points and Methods
3–4 U is injected 1 cm lateral to the midline along the mandible at each side. 1–2 U is injected shallowly 1–2 cm superior to the jaw line and 1 cm lateral to the midline at each

side (Fig. 2.39). Injecting too laterally from the midline of the mandible may involve the depressor labii inferioris m., which would lead to a dysfunctional mouth with a ptosis of the lower lip.

2.2.14 Platysmal Band

The platysmal band, considered another target for botulinum toxin treatment, can be caused by changes in the length of the platysma muscle when aging. This wrinkle can be observed as vertical lines from the jaw line to the neck area when speaking or even staying still (Fig. 2.40a). Normally, the platysma draws down the modiolus, the corners of the mouth, and the lower cheek, pulling down the lower region of the face and inferolaterally pulling the mouth corner. Therefore, when it repeatedly contracts, it contributes to aging symptoms and signs, such as a drooping of the mouth corner and jowl sagging. Fat deposits and skin laxity in the medial and lateral border of the platysma cause the "gobbler neck deformity," easily found in western seniors.

Fig. 2.38 The location of the mentalis muscle origin and insertion (**a**). Medial fibers of the mentalis forming a dome-shaped chin prominence in the posterior aspect. In this view, the medial fibers of the mentalis descend anteromedially to cross together, thus forming a dome-shaped chin prominence (**b**). *OM* medial border of origin, *OL* distal border of origin, *IM* medial border of insertion, *IL* lateral border of insertion (Published with kind permission of © Hee-Jin Kim and Kwan-Hyun Youn 2016. All rights reserved)

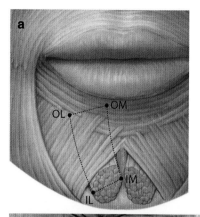

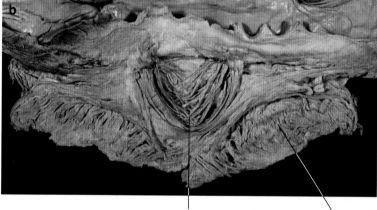

Mentalis m.   Depressor labii inferioris m.

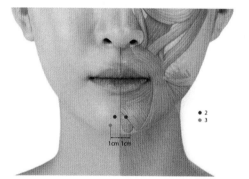

Fig. 2.39 Injection points of botulinum toxin for cobble stone chin (Published with kind permission of © Kwan-Hyun Youn 2016. All rights reserved)

2.2.14.1 Target Muscle and Anatomy

The platysma, which is the thinning of the subcutaneous muscle, arises from the fascia of the deltoid and the pectoralis major m., extends over the clavicle, and covers the entire neck and lower face. Most muscle fibers extend over the mandible and run deeper into the inner face than the modiolus, the DAO, and the risorius muscle. However, some of them attach to the mandible. In the cheek, the platysma runs upward, continuing with the SMAS layer and covering the masseter muscle and the parotid gland (Fig. 2.40b).

2.2.14.2 Injection Points and Methods
(Fig. 2.42)

When the entire platysma is in action, it draws the corner of the mouth inferiorly and laterally. Botulinum toxin is injected into the platysma when acting from the inferior border of the mandible to the clavicle. 2 U is injected per point, and injection points are placed for each band approximately 1.5–2 cm from each other along the muscular band. The standard dosage for Asians is 10–20 U at each muscular band, and the total dose should not exceed 50 U.

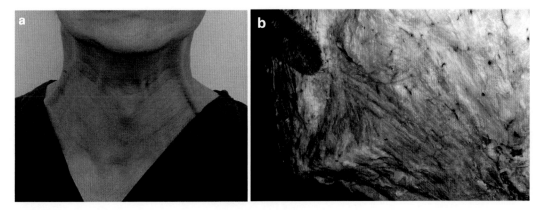

Fig. 2.40 Platysmal band (**a**) and insertion of the platysma muscle into the lower face (**b**) (Published with kind permission of © Kyle K Seo and Hee-Jin Kim 2016. All rights reserved)

Decussation Patterns of the Platysma in Asians (Fig. 2.41)

There are no platysma muscle fibers in the superficial layer of the mid-neck area. Some fibers are decussated and interlaced at the upper anterior neck, covering the submental region. In Asians, 85 % of bilateral medial platysmal fibers are interlaced at the submental region. And, in particular, 43 % showed decussation over 20 mm below the chin. On the other hand, non-decussation patterns were much more frequent in Caucasians (39 %) than in Asians (15 %). These findings may explain why Asians have a lower incidence of the "gobbler neck deformity" than Caucasians.

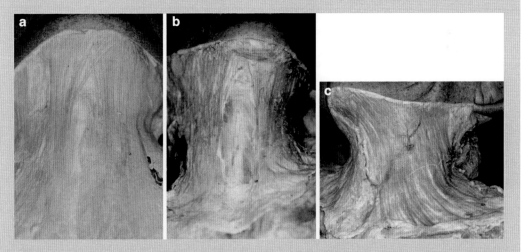

Fig. 2.41 Platysmal patterns in Korean. Bilateral medial platysmal fibers interlaced at the submental region (**a** decussation pattern) in 85 % of the specimens. In 15 % of the cases, they did not (**b** non-decussation pattern). (**c**) Lateral aspect of the dissection of the platysma (Published with kind permission of © Hee-Jin Kim 2016. All rights reserved)

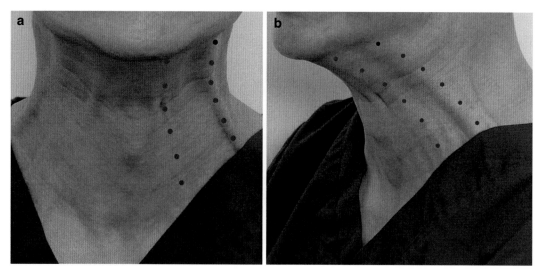

Fig. 2.42 Injection points of botulinum toxin for platysmal band (*violet* and *black dots*) (**a** frontal view, **b** lateral view) (Published with kind permission of © Kyle K Seo 2016. All rights reserved)

2.3   Botulinum Facial Contouring

2.3.1   Masseter Hypertrophy
(Fig. 2.43)

2.3.1.1 Target Muscle and Anatomy
The masseter arises from the zygomatic arch, runs along the mandibular angle obliquely and inferoposteriorly, and attaches to the mandibular angle and the ramus of the mandible (Fig. 2.44). It consists of three layers according to depth. The superficial portion arises from the zygomatic process of the maxilla, and, from the anterior two-thirds of the lower border of the zygomatic arch, it runs posteriorly and inserts into the masseteric tuberosity on the outer surface of the mandibular ramus around the mandibular angle. The middle portion originates from the deep surface of the anterior two-thirds of the zygomatic arch, and, from the lower border of the posterior one-third of the arch, it runs vertically and inserts on the upper and lateral surface of the ramus. The deepest portion, also known as the zygomaticomandibularis m., arises from the deep surface of the zygomatic arch and attaches to the middle part of the ramus. The masseteric n., a branch of the mandibular n., passes between the middle and deep layer of the masseter and separates the middle layer from the deep layer of the masseter

(Fig. 2.45). The superficial layer is the largest, and three layers of the muscle fibers are overlaid, forming the thickest layer at the lower portion. Therefore, the botulinum toxin injection should be performed into the lower portion, where the area is the thickest.

Cross-sectional areas and volumes of the masseter were measured from CT scans of 65 Chinese. Idiopathic masseter muscle hypertrophy patients recorded 1.3 cm, though normal instances record 0.8 cm. When measuring masseters using 3D CT scans for 28 Korean women, the depth of the lower border was 34.7 ± 3.2 mm (25.0–40.0 mm), and the thickness was 14.9 ± 2.2 mm (10.6–20.1 mm) (unpublished materials).

2.3.1.2 Injection Points and Methods
Injections should be deeply made into the lower 1/3 of the masseter at four injection points. A shallow toxin injection into the masseter m. causes a change in facial expression, with the most frequently reported change being a reduction in the width of the mouth upon smiling. This is because the toxin spreads into the risorius m. located in front of the masseter. The line connection lobule and the cheilion are references and divide into superior and inferior masseters. The injection points are located below this line. Injection points are placed inferior to

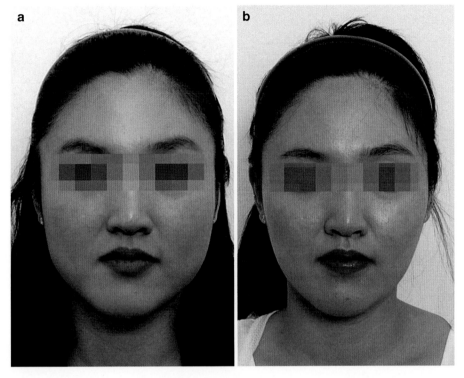

Fig. 2.43 Before (**a**) and after (**b**) of botulinum toxin injection for the masseter hypertrophy (Published with kind permission of © Kyle K Seo 2016. All rights reserved)

Fig. 2.44 Masseter muscle (Published with kind permission of © Kwan-Hyun Youn 2016. All rights reserved)

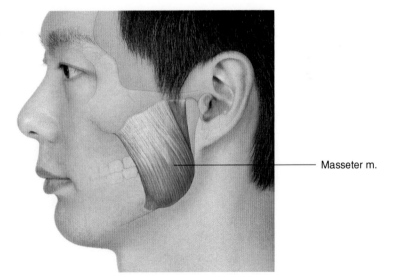

Masseter m.

the masseter because it has well-developed muscle fibers and is the most prominent area. Additionally, cheekbones appear more prominent due to atrophy of the lower part of the cheekbone when injections are made into the upper area, especially for Koreans with high cheekbones. With respect to toxin injections into the masseter, clinicians delineate a safe

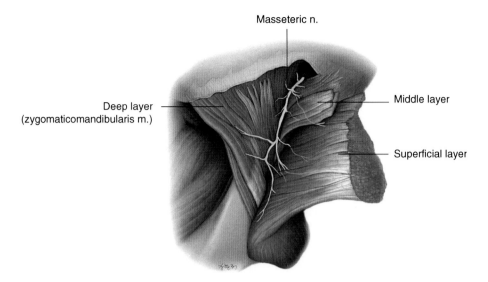

Masseteric n.

Deep layer
(zygomaticomandibularis m.)

Middle layer

Superficial layer

Fig. 2.45   Three layers of the masseter muscle and innervating masseteric nerve (Published with kind permission of © Kwan-Hyun Youn 2016. All rights reserved)

Fig. 2.46   Injection points of botulinum
toxin for masseter hypertrophy
(Published with kind permission of
© Kwan-Hyun Youn 2016. All rights
reserved)

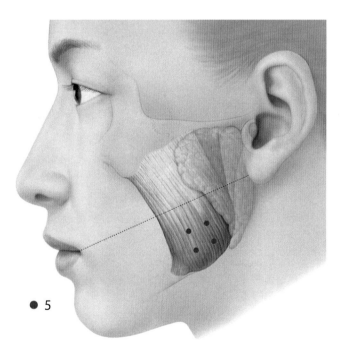

● 5

injection zone using four lines: two lines of the anterior and posterior margins of the masseter muscle, one line connecting the earlobe and the mouth corner, and one line within 1 cm of the mandibular border.

10–40 U is injected at each side, depending on the volume of the masseter. 20 U is enough for a width and thickness of 3–5 cm. As an exception, 25–40 U could be injected for a man with a width of over 5 cm or thicker (Fig. 2.46).

Precautions of the Position of the Risorius During Botulinum Facial Contouring

A shallow toxin injection into the masseter m. when contouring the lower face causes asymmetric smiles, with the most frequently reported change being a reduction in the width of the mouth upon smiling. These could be explained by the degree of toxin diffusion depending on the amount and location of the toxin injection. This is because the toxin spreads into the risorius m., located in front of the masseter.

Anatomy of the risorius m.: The risorius m. is very thin and is located 20–50 mm lateral to the cheilion and 0–15 mm inferior to the intercheilion horizontal line. It arises from the SMAS (superficial musculoaponeurotic system), the parotid fascia, the masseteric fascia, the platysma, and, in rare cases, from the tendon of masseter muscle. It originates from multiple layers and inserts into the modiolus. Its functions are to pull the mouth corners superiorly and laterally when smiling. It plays an important role with the zygomaticus major when grinning. If the toxin spreads into the neighboring risorius m. when injected into the

surface of masseter, it can cause changes in facial expression.

This muscle generally arises from 1/3 anterior or, in rare cases, 2/3 anterior to the masseter surface on the SMAS layer. A well-developed risorius m. passes the fascia of the masseter and covers the lateral face until it is superior to the parotid gland (Fig. 2.47).

Someone with a well-developed risorius m. moves the ears upward or backward when smiling broadly. It is reasonable to assume that the platysma, which is the same layer as the risorius, crosses over the zygomatic arch and becomes continuous with the temporoparietal fascia and the auricular muscle. This causes the ears to move when the risorius and the SMAS move.

Prevention: To prevent toxin from diffusing into the risorius after injection into the masseter, the needle is injected deeply into the masseter until the tip is just above the mandibular surface. In particular, the recommended dosage for someone with a well-developed risorius is under 10 U at each side to avoid toxin diffusion on the masseter surface.

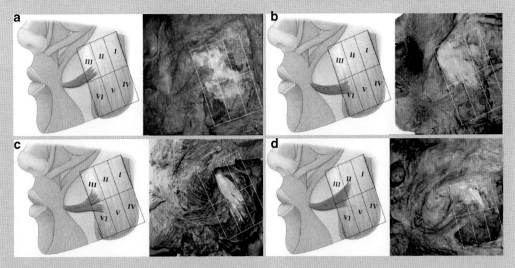

Fig. 2.47 Classification of the relationship between the risorius and masseter muscle. (**a**) The risorius muscle covers area III; (**b**) the risorius muscle covers area VI; (**c**) the risorius muscle covers areas III *and* VI; and (**d**) the risorius muscle covers areas II, III, and VI (Published with kind permission of © Hee-Jin Kim and Kwan-Hyun Youn 2016. All rights reserved)

2.3.2 Temporalis Hypertrophy

2.3.2.1 Target Muscle and Anatomy

Botulinum treatment can be used in cases when the upper face appears wider and the muscle appears prominent. This is because the temporalis m. is well developed (Fig. 2.48).

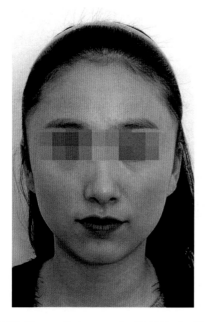

Fig. 2.48 Temporalis hypertrophy (Published with kind permission of © Kyle K Seo 2016. All rights reserved)

This muscle is flat and fan shaped and consists of two layers. The superficial layer arises from the temporal fascia, and most of the deep layers arise from the bone around the temporal fossa. Most of the origin is composed of the muscular belly, and the middle portion is composed of the tendon, which is attached to the coronoid process. The anterior part runs almost vertically, whereas the posterior portion runs almost horizontally. The temporal fascia covering the surface of this muscle is strong fascia. The upper part of this muscle is attached to the superior temporal line, and the lower part is attached to the upper margin of the zygomatic arch (Fig. 2.49). The anterior, middle, and posterior deep temporal n. is innervated, and the anterior and posterior deep temporal arteries are distributed in the temporalis. It acts to elevate the mandible and to close the mouth. It also acts to keep the tension maintenance against the gravity and to maintain a closed-mouth position.

2.3.2.2 Injection Points and Methods

20–40 U is injected into the developed muscle and divided into four to six parts. The injection site is the upper 1/2 of the temporalis because the upper area is more protrusive and more involved

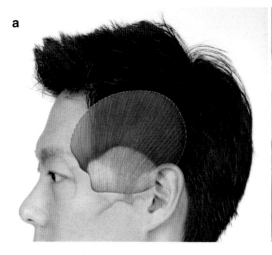

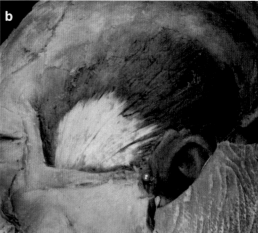

Fig. 2.49 Temporalis muscle (**a**, **b**) (Published with kind permission of © Hee-Jin Kim and Kwan-Hyun Youn 2016. All rights reserved)

in the size of the face. Clinicians should take care when injecting into this muscle because an excess of toxin may result in a sunken shape (Fig. 2.50).

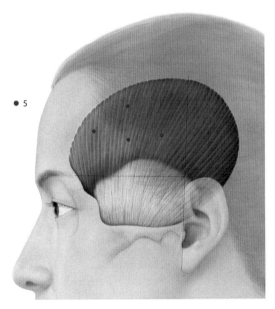

● 5

Fig. 2.50 Injection points of botulinum toxin for temporalis hypertrophy (Published with kind permission of © Kwan-Hyun Youn 2016. All rights reserved)

2.3.3 Hypertrophy of the Salivary Gland (Figs. 2.51 and 2.52)

2.3.3.1 Target Muscle and Anatomy (Figs. 2.53 and 2.54)

A well-developed parotid gland situated posterolaterally to the masseter prevents the effect of treatments for masseter hypertrophy despite a decreased volume of the masseter. In this case, injecting into the parotid gland with the masseter can decrease the volume of the parotid gland. Therefore, the face can become slimmer.

This gland is situated on the posterior border of the mandible, which includes the mandibular angle. It is divided into superficial and deep layers. The superficial layer is located on the masseter fascia, and the deep layer covers the masseter and the mandible since it is placed on the medial side covering the mandibular ramus.

Some patients who had undergone angle reduction complained that the bulging in the neck area is due to a well-developed submandibular gland. In this case, direct toxin injection into the submandibular area can reduce the volume of the gland as well. The submandibular gland is situated inferior and superior to the submandibular triangle, producing the most amount of saliva. Patients, therefore, complain of xerostomia.

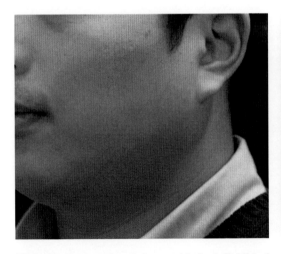

Fig. 2.51 Hypertrophy of the parotid gland (Published with kind permission of © Hong-Ki Lee 2016. All rights reserved)

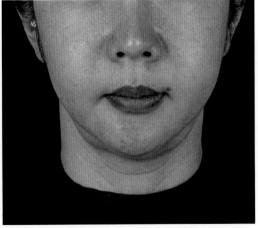

Fig. 2.52 Hypertrophy of the submandibular gland (Published with kind permission of © Gee-Young Bae and Kyle K Seo 2016. All rights reserved)

Fig. 2.53 Parotid gland
(Published with kind
permission of © Hee-Jin
Kim 2016. All rights
reserved)

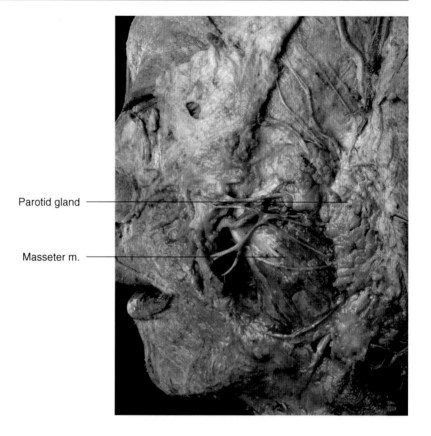

Parotid gland ——

Masseter m. ——

Fig. 2.54 Submandibular
gland (Published with kind
permission of © Hee-Jin
Kim 2016. All rights
reserved)

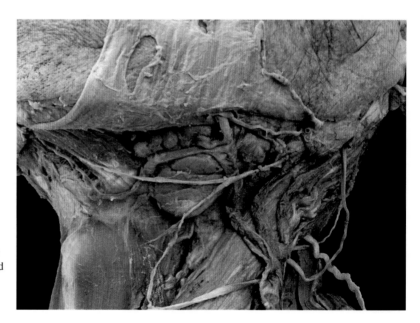

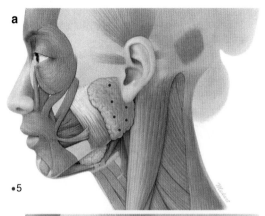

a

•5

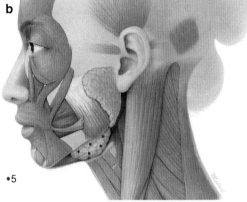

b

•5

Fig. 2.55 Injection points of botulinum toxin for hypertrophy of the parotid gland (**a**) and submandibular gland (**b**) (Published with kind permission of © Kwan-Hyun Youn 2016. All rights reserved)

2.3.3.2 Injection Points and Methods

The botulinum toxin dose for the parotid gland is 30 U at each side, divided into four to five injection points. 20–30 U is injected into the submandibular gland (Fig. 2.55).

Suggested Reading

Muscles of the Face and Neck

1. Bae JH, Choi DY, Lee JG, Tansatit T, Kim HJ. The risorius muscle: anatomic considerations with reference to botulinum neurotoxin injection for masseteric hypertrophy. Dermatol Surg. 2014;40(12):1334–9.
2. Bae JH, Lee JH, Youn KH, Hur MS, Hu KS, Tansatit T, Kim HJ. Surgical consideration of the anatomic origin of the risorius in relation to facial planes. Aesthet Surg. 2014;34:JNP43–9.
3. Choi DY, Kim JS, Youn KH, Hur MS, Kim JS, Hu KS, Kim HJ. Clinical anatomic considerations of the zygomaticus minor muscle based on the morphology and insertion pattern. Dermatol Surg. 2014;40(8):858–63.
4. Choi YJ, Kim JS, Gil YC, Phetudom T, Kim HJ, Tansatit T, Hu KS. Anatomic considerations regarding the location and boundary of the depressor anguli oris muscle with reference to botulinum toxin injection. Plast Reconstr Surg. 2014;134(5):917–21.
5. Hu KS, Jin GC, Youn KH, Kwak HH, Koh KS, Fontaine C, Kim HJ. An anatomic study of the bifid zygomaticus major muscle. J Craniofac Surg. 2008;19(2):534–5.
6. Hu KS, Kim ST, Hur MS, Park JH, Song WC, Koh KS, Kim HJ. Topography of the masseter muscle in relation to treatment with botulinum toxin type A. Oral Surg Oral Med O. 2010;110(2):167–71.
7. Hur MS, Hu KS, Cho JY, Kwak HH, Song WC, Koh KS, Lorente M, Kim HJ. Topography and location of the depressor anguli oris muscle with a reference to the mental foramen. Surg Radiol Anat. 2008;30(5):403–7.
8. Hur MS, Hu KS, Kwak HH, Lee KS, Kim HJ. Inferior bundle (fourth band) of the buccinators and the incisivus labii inferioris muscle. J Craniofac Surg. 2011;22(1):289–92.
9. Hur MS, Hu KS, Park JT, Youn KH, Kim HJ. New anatomical insight of the levator labii superioris alaeque nasi and the transverse part of the nasalis. Surg Radiol Anat. 2010;32(8):753–6.
10. Hur MS, Hu KS, Youn KH, Song WC, Abe S, Kim HJ. New anatomical profile of the nasal musculature: dilator naris vestibularis, dilator naris anterior, and alar part of the nasalis. Clin Anat. 2011;24(2):162–7.
11. Hur MS, Kim HJ, Choi BY, Hu KS, Kim HJ, Lee KS. Morphology of the mentalis muscle and its relationship with the orbicularis oris and incisivus labii inferioris muscles. J Craniofac Surg. 2013;24(2):602–4.
12. Hur MS, Youn KH, Hu KS, Song WC, Koh KS, Fontaine C, Kim HJ. New anatomic considerations on the levator labii superioris related with the nasal ala. J Craniofac Surg. 2010;21(1):258–60.
13. Hwang WS, Hur MS, Hu KS, Song WC, Koh KS, Baik HS, Kim ST, Kim HJ, Lee KJ. Surface anatomy of the lip elevator muscles for the treatment of gummy smile using botulinum toxin. Angle Orthod. 2009;79(1):70–7.
14. Kim HJ, Hu KS, Kang MK, Hwang K, Chung IH. Decussation patterns of the platysma in Koreans. Br J Plast Surg. 2001;54(5):400–2.
15. Kim HS, Pae C, Bae JH, Hu KS, Chang BM, Tansatit T, Kim HJ. An anatomical study of the risorius in Asians and its insertion at the modiolus. Surg Radiol Anat. 2014;37(2):147–51.
16. Lee JY, Kim JN, Kim SH, Choi HG, Hu KS, Kim HJ, Song WC, Koh KS. Anatomical verification and designation of the superficial layer of the temporalis muscle. Clin Anat. 2012;25(2):176–81.
17. Lee JY, Kim JN, Yoo JY, Hu KS, Kim HJ, Song WC, Koh KS. Topographic anatomy of the masseter mus-

cle focusing on the tendinous digitation. Clin Anat. 2012;25(7):889–92.

18. Park JT, Youn KH, Hu KS, Kim HJ. Medial muscular band of the orbicularis oculi muscle. J Craniofac Surg. 2012;23(1):195–7.

19. Park JT, Youn KH, Hur MS, Hu KS, Kim HJ, Kim HJ. Malaris muscle, the lateral muscular band of orbicularis oculi muscle. J Craniofac Surg. 2011;22(2):659–62.

20. Shim KS, Hu KS, Kwak HH, Youn KH, Koh KS, Fontaine C, Kim HJ. An anatomy of the insertion of the zygomaticus major muscle in human focused on the muscle arrangement at the mouth corner. Plast Reconstr Surg. 2008;121(2):466–73.

21. Yang HM, Kim HJ. Anatomical study of the corrugator supercilii muscle and its clinical implication with botulinum toxin A injection. Surg Radiol Anat. 2013;35(9):817–21.

22. Youn KH, Park JT, Park DS, Koh KS, Kim HJ, Paik DJ. Morphology of the zygomaticus minor and its relationship with the orbicularis oculi muscle. J Craniofac Surg. 2012;23(2):546–8.

23. Yu SK, Lee MH, Kim HS, Park JT, Kim HJ, Kim HJ. Histomorphologic approach for the modiolus with reference to reconstructive and aesthetic surgery. J Craniofac Surg. 2013;24(4):1414–7.

Peripheral Nerves of the Face and Neck

24. Kim DH, Hong HS, Won SY, Kim HJ, Hu KS, Choi JH, Kim HJ. Intramuscular nerve distribution of the masseter muscle for botulinum toxin injection. J Craniofac Surg. 2010;21(2):588–91.

25. Kwak HH, Ko SJ, Jung HS, Park HD, Chung IH, Kim HJ. Topographic anatomy of the deep temporal nerves, with references to the superior head of lateral pterygoid. Surg Radiol Anat. 2003;25(5–6):393–9.

26. Kwak HH, Park HD, Youn KH, Hu KS, Koh KS, Han SH, Kim HJ. Branching patterns of the facial nerve and its communication with the auriculotemporal nerve. Surg Radiol Anat. 2004;26(6):494–500.

27. Won SY, Kim DH, Yang HM, Park JT, Kwak HH, Hu KS, Kim HJ. Clinical and anatomical approach using Sihler's staining technique (whole mount nerve stain). Anat Cell Biol. 2011;44(1):1–7.

28. Yang HM, Won SY, Kim HJ, Hu KS. Sihler staining study of anastomosis between the facial and trigeminal nerves in the ocular area and its clinical implications. Muscle Nerve. 2013;48(4):545–50.

Others

29. Carruthers ACJ. Botulinum toxin. Elsevier Science Health Science div. 2013;3:52–8.

30. Dessy LA, Mazzocchi M, Rubino C, Mazzarello V, Spissu N, Scuderi N. An objective assessment of botulinum toxin A effect on superficial skin texture. Ann Plast Surg. 2007;58(5):469–73.

31. Flynn TC, Carruthers JA, Carruthers JA. Botulinum-A toxin treatment of the lower eyelid improves infraorbital rhytides and widens the eye. Dermatol Surg. 2001;27(8):703–8.

32. Frankel AS, Kamer FM. Chemical browlift. Arch Otolaryngol Head Neck Surg. 2007;124(3):321–3.

33. Huilgol SC, Carruthers A, Carruthers JD. Raising eyebrows with botulinum toxin. Dermatol Surg. 1999;25(5):373–5.

34. Kyle K. Seo: Botulinum treatment. Seoul Medical Publishing Co. 2014;2:182–3.

35. Xu JA, Yuasa K, Yoshiura K, Kanda S. Quantitative analysis of masticatory muscles using computed tomography. Dentomaxillofac Radiol. 1994;23(3):154–8.

Clinical Anatomy of the Upper Face for Filler Injection

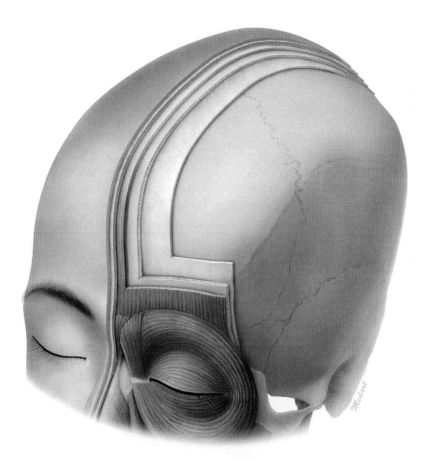

Hong-Ki Lee, MD, PhD, Jisoo Kim, MD, MS, Hee-Jin Kim, DDS, PhD (Illustrated by Kwan-Hyun Youn)

© Springer Science+Business Media Singapore 2016
H.-J. Kim et al., *Clinical Anatomy of the Face for Filler and Botulinum Toxin Injection*,
DOI 10.1007/978-981-10-0240-3_3

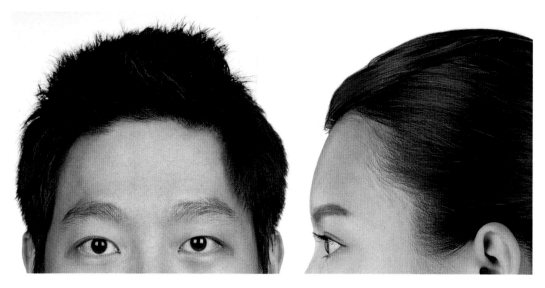

Fig. 3.1 Surface contour of the forehead and glabella (Published with kind permission of © Kwan-Hyun Youn 2016. All rights reserved)

3.1　Forehead and Glabella

The hairline and eyebrows form demarcations superior and inferior to the forehead, respectively. An undulated forehead may give an aging impression; therefore, fat grafting and filler injection are often used as cosmetic treatments to improve uneven surface of the forehead into convex and smooth ones. Cosmetic filler injections are often used to create a smooth and convex curvature from the trichion to the eyebrow (Fig. 3.1). In contrast to the dolichocephalic-type skull predominant in white populations, the brachycephalic-type skull is predominant in Asian populations. A smooth and convex forehead allows the entire face to look smaller, which satisfies the aesthetic demand of Asian populations.

Cosmetic filler treatment can be used to diminish the appearance of a more pronounced glabellar frown line, often resulting from continual frowning, and to make up for a loss of volume near the glabellar area, often resulting from aging.

3.1.1　Clinical Anatomy

A naturally wide concavity is commonly located between the frontal eminence and the supercili-ary arch; however, there are cases in which the center of the forehead or the area above the lateral eyebrow is partially sunken. These areas must also be identified prior to treatment. Furthermore, the concave area from the point "metopion (midpoint between the frontal eminence of the forehead)" to the superciliary arch must be laterally identified (Fig. 3.2).

The forehead is wide, and the soft tissue is thin (<2 mm). Fat atrophy occurs both congenitally and after birth, resulting in the accentuation of bone structure, which gives the appearance of aging. In this case, the shape of the forehead may be rough and uneven; therefore, the sunken areas must be identified. The forehead is composed of the skin-subcutaneous tissue-frontalis m. with the galea aponeurosis-loose connective tissue-periosteum of the frontal bone. The frontalis m. is very thin and the subcutaneous fat composition in the forehead is low (Fig. 3.3).

3.1.2　Injection Points and Methods

The forehead is a highly sensitive area; therefore, nerve block is necessary prior to filler injection. The supraorbital n. and the supra-trochlear n. traversing the forehead must be anesthetized (refer to the topic of anesthetic

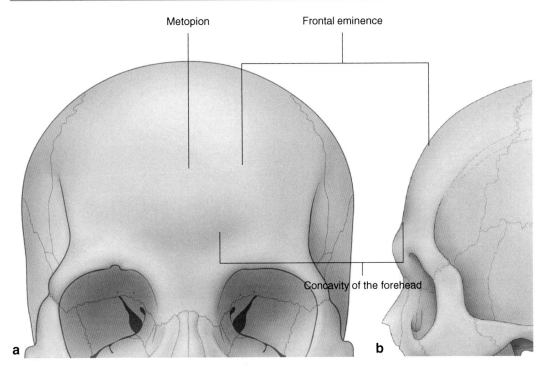

Fig. 3.2 Frontal eminence and the concavity of the forehead (**a** frontal view, **b** lateral view) (Published with kind permission of © Kwan-Hyun Youn 2016. All rights reserved)

methods in Chap. 1). When treating the lateral side of the forehead, the zygomaticotemporal n. may also need to be anesthetized. Direct local infiltration in this area is preferred due to the incomplete nerve block of the zygomaticotemporal nerve (Fig. 3.4).

Supraperiosteal injection into the loose connective tissue layer is preffered for safety and surface irregularity (Fig. 3.3). Because the forehead area is wide, there is a high probability of irregular bulging due to thin surface level, and it is difficult to raise its volume. Additionally, it is recommended that injections above the periosteum to avoid injecting into the branched arteries and veins of the forehead that run along the superficial layer of the forehead.

For more pronounced and general depression at glabellar frown lines, injection above the periosteum is preferable. However, when glabellar frown lines are slight, superficial injection into the subdermal layer can be effective to eliminate the dermal crease.

During injections to the forehead, it is difficult to avoid every vessel; therefore, to treat the forehead is strongly advice to use a cannula. Even if the cannula is used to inject above the periosteum, safety is not 100% guaranteed. Furthermore, extra caution must be taken into consideration to avoid arteries passing through the bone to the skin and other areas where vessels branch out. A possible method is to inject after first inserting the cannula into the target area and waiting to see if hematoma occurs. When using a cannula of too small caliber, excessive pressure may result in a punctured vein; therefore, a cannula of around 23–25 G is recommended.

When determining the entry point of the cannula, it is recommended that the area where the superficial temporal a. passes the lateral border of the frontalis m. and the area where the supraorbital a. branches out should be avoided. The area 2 cm above the eyebrow in the longitudinal plane of the lateral canthus is where the frontal branch of the superficial temporal a. passes. It is possible to avoid the artery within a 2 cm superior from the lateral canthus with approaching from the lateral border of the forehead (Fig. 3.5).

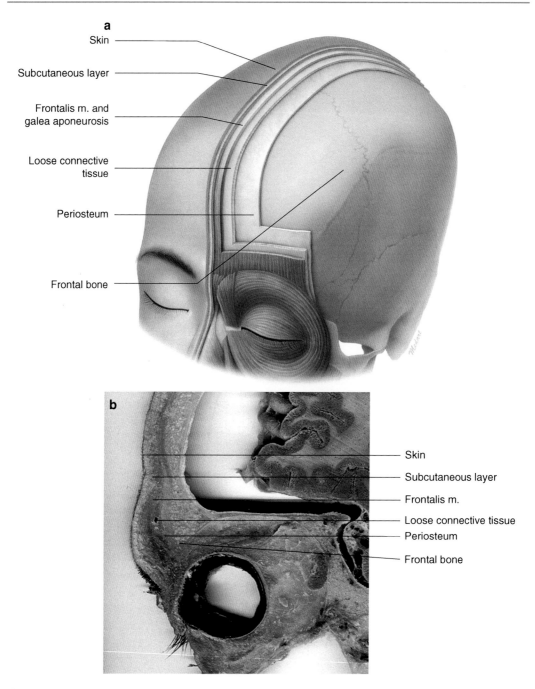

Fig. 3.3 Anatomical layers of the forehead and glabella (**a**, **b**) (Published with kind permission of © Hee-Jin Kim and Kwan-Hyun Youn 2016. All rights reserved)

The most common cannula injection point is located at borders between the forehead and the temporal region. Furthermore, the metopion of the median line of the forehead can serve as an injection point due to its relatively unpronounced vessel dispersion (Fig. 3.6a). In the case where the curvature of the metopion is too angular, it is difficult to inject below the muscle layer at the point of the angular curvature. In this case, the injection point should be placed at the medial

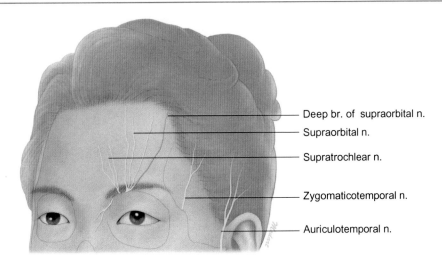

Fig. 3.4 Nerve innervations on the forehead and temple (Published with kind permission of © Kwan-Hyun Youn 2016. All rights reserved)

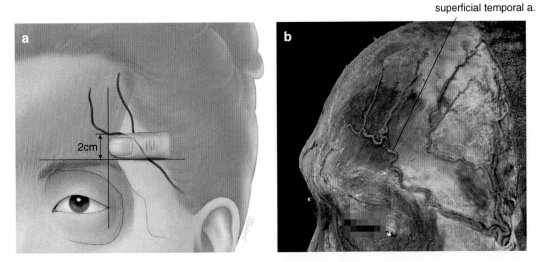

Fig. 3.5 Frontal branch of the superficial temporal artery passing the lateral border of the frontalis muscle (**a, b**) (Published with kind permission of © Hee-Jin Kim and Kwan-Hyun Youn 2016. All rights reserved)

corner of the eyebrow, and the cannula should be inserted below the muscle layer (Fig. 3.6b). Even when using the cannula as an injection tool, the cannula must be placed below the muscle layer and above the periosteum. The injection must proceed as the cannula is slowly retrogradely from its position (Figs. 3.7 and 3.8).

When the area is partially dented or sunken, it is possible to use a needle. If possible, it is advised that the needle be inserted through the muscle layer until the point where the tip of the needle touches the bone. After it is made certain that the needle touches the bone, the filler should be injected above the periosteum in small volume. Massaging the area of injection and allowing the filler to spread throughout the loose connective tissue layer can prevent undulations on the surface. Direct filler injections to the vessel can be confirmed by aspiration prior to injection. The use of a cannula is recommended when injecting the area where the supraorbital and supratrochlear a. branches out.

Filler treatments on the glabella pose the highest risk for visual loss among patients due to embolism and intravascular injection; therefore,

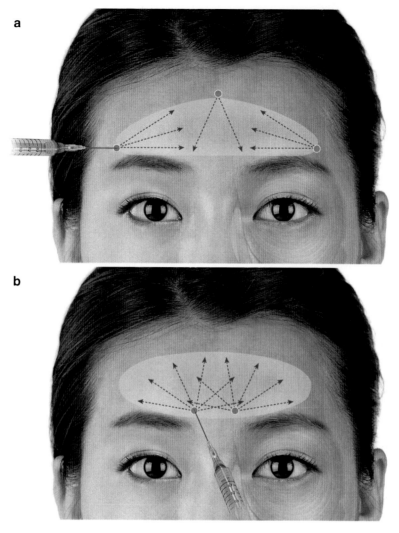

Fig. 3.6 Filler injection techniques for the forehead using cannula ((**a**) lateral approach, (**b**) medial approach) (Published with kind permission of © Kwan-Hyun Youn 2016. All rights reserved)

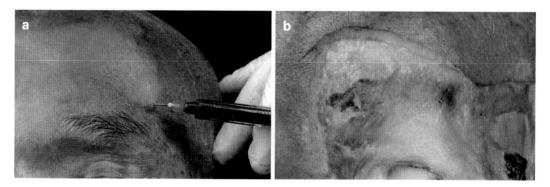

Fig. 3.7 Filler injection on the cadaveric forehead using cannula (**a**) and the properly located filler product beneath the frontalis muscle (**b**) (Published with kind permission of © Hee-Jin Kim 2016. All rights reserved)

Fig. 3.8 Safe injection plane of filler on the forehead and glabella (Published with kind permission of © Kwan-Hyun Youn 2016. All rights reserved)

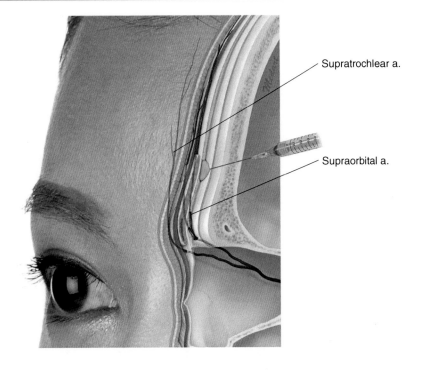

Supratrochlear a.

Supraorbital a.

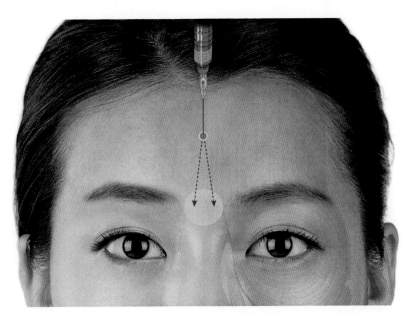

Fig. 3.9 Filler injection technique for the glabella using cannula (Published with kind permission of © Kwan-Hyun Youn 2016. All rights reserved)

the use of a cannula is highly recommended. When using a needle, the soft tissue of this area is lifted in order to allow injection into the subdermis in small quantities. Another method is to insert the needle so that it touches the bone and to inject the filler in small quantities. The insertion of the cannula should proceed from the middle of the forehead (Fig. 3.9).

3.1.3   Side Effects

Skin necrosis of the forehead may occur due to lack of blood circulation, and special caution must be taken with regard to branching of vessels and tissue layers. The arteries to be treated with caution are the supratrochlear a., the supraorbital a., and the frontal branch of the superficial temporal artery (Figs. 3.5 and 3.10). The supraorbital a. traverses the supraorbital foramen or notch, while the supratrochlear a. passes through the orbital septum and up the forehead through the muscle and subcutaneous tissue layers. Therefore, it is advised that, when conducting filler treatments on the forehead, the cannula be placed and injected along the supraperiosteal layer. It also follows that special caution must be taken to avoid damaging blood vessels traversing the supraorbital foramen or notch and the inner eye area when inserting a needle or cannula close to the periosteum. Even the use of a cannula runs the risk of damaging blood vessels and nerves; therefore, the filler injection should be conducted

slowly while staying alert for the presence of hematomas. Since veins have a larger diameter and a weaker wall, veins are still susceptible to damage and contusion even with the use of a cannula. Thus, it is pivotal that the injection is made slowly and gently.

Injection of large amount of fillers into the lateral side of the forehead can lead to engorged veins due to increased local pressure. Extra caution must be taken during the filler injection if the patient possesses bulging veins on target area.

Glabellar wrinkles that have become static wrinkles are difficult to be corrected. In such cases, a needle is used to inject the filler directly into the subcutaneous or muscle layer, while the injection path follows the path of the wrinkle. In actuality, the supratrochlear a. travels closer to the surface than the adjacent supraorbital a. When injecting fillers into this area via a needle, the risk of the filler spreading throughout the dermis and causing damage to the supratrochlear a. must be taken into consideration.

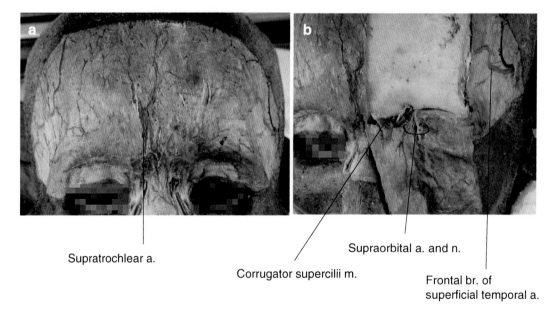

Supratrochlear a.

Corrugator supercilii m.

Supraorbital a. and n.

Frontal br. of superficial temporal a.

Fig. 3.10 Blood supply of the forehead and glabella (**a**, **b**) (Published with kind permission of © Hee-Jin Kim 2016. All rights reserved)

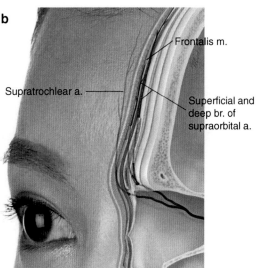

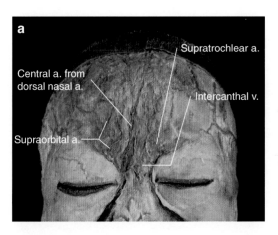

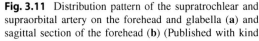

Fig. 3.11 Distribution pattern of the supratrochlear and supraorbital artery on the forehead and glabella (**a**) and sagittal section of the forehead (**b**) (Published with kind permission of © Hee-Jin Kim and Kwan-Hyun Youn 2016. All rights reserved)

Furthermore, there is also the danger of intravascular injection of the filler into the supratrochlear artery. Even if the injection is placed at the subcutaneous layer, a brash injection may damage the subdermal vascular plexus, resulting in local skin necrosis. In order to avoid an increase of local pressure in the dermis, the injection must be performed slowly and with caution (Figs. 3.11 and 3.13).

The use of a cannula is advised since it precludes the possibility of intravascular injection. Moreover, excessive use of fillers or the use of hydrophilic fillers poses a risk of attracting water, which results in swelling and increase local pressure. Overall, when reducing glabellar frown lines via filler injection, special care must be taken to avoid the supratrochlear a. that runs through the glabella region (Fig. 3.11).

Moreover, contact with the supraorbital n. during injection will lead to the patient feeling pain throughout his or her vertex or occipital region. In order to avoid any unnecessary pain, it is advised that the cannula be placed closer to the periosteum.

Tip: Forehead Filler Injection When conducting filler injections on the forehead, it is better to focus on creating smooth curvatures rather than on increasing volume (Fig. 3.12). The forehead—being a large, thin area—can easily form undulations when not treated with care. In order to avoid undulations, injecting fillers into periosteal level with smooth properties is advised as it also helps to avoid the danger of intravascular injection.

A cannula is often used when inserting fillers into the forehead; however, it is not easy to continuously follow the curvature of the forehead while maintaining tip of cannula on the periosteum. If the curvature of the forehead is not taken into consideration and filler injections made obliquely with a straight cannula, a large proportion of the filler may be inserted into the subcutaneous layer. Even if the cannula initially touched the periosteum, the cannula

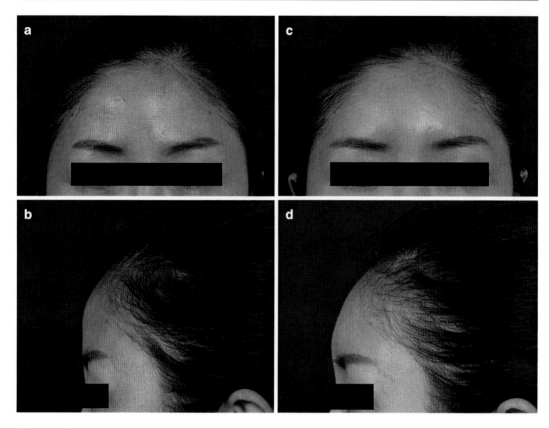

Fig. 3.12 Forehead augmentation using filler before (**a**, **b**) and after (**c**, **d**) the injection (Published with kind permission of © Hong-Ki Lee 2016. All rights reserved)

may move from its original position following the curvature of the forehead and into the subcutaneous layer (Fig. 3.13). In order to avoid the abovementioned case, the length of the cannula and the curvature of the forehead must be taken into consideration prior to insertion. Furthermore, multiple insertion points must be confirmed, and the cannula should be inserted through the muscle layer and touch the periosteum. Injection should proceed with uniform pressure and volume. It is recommended to use a flexible cannula with a size ranging between 23 and 25 G.

Tip: Glabella Filler Injection Wrinkles can generally be categorized into two groups: static wrinkles and dynamic wrinkles. Botulinum toxin is commonly used to treat wrinkles according to muscle movement. Nonetheless, in the case of static wrinkles, filler treatment may be necessary. Fine wrinkles may be reduced by filler injection into the dermis or subdermis. The appearance of deeper wrinkles may be reduced by substituting volume via filler injection. The constant movement of dynamic wrinkles may lead to filler migration; therefore, filler injection should be carried out with crossing technique, rather than running along the line.

Fig. 3.13 Dangerous
injection plane of filler on
the forehead and glabella
(Published with kind
permission of © Kwan-
Hyun Youn 2016. All
rights reserved)

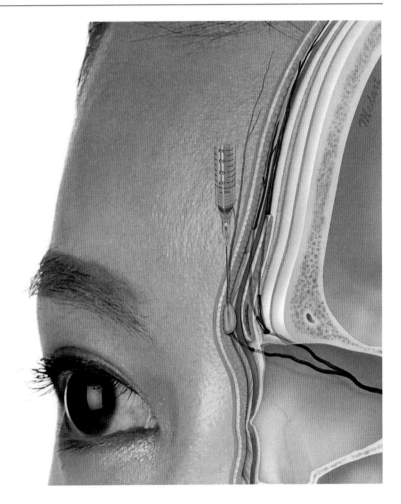

3.2   Sunken Eye and Pretarsal Roll

The depression of the upper eyelid region may
occur congenitally or occur because of aging,
giving off a tired and elderly appearance. For
Asians, the presence of a pretarsal roll gives a
younger and cuter appearance of eyes when smiling (Fig. 3.14).

3.2.1   Clinical Anatomy

The eyelid and orbital region comprise of the
upper eyelid (the area above the palpebral fissure and below the eyebrow), the medial canthus (the medial point where the upper and
lower eyelids fuse), the later canthus (the lateral
point where the upper and lower eyelids fuse),
and the lower eyelid (the area below the palpebral fissure). Although they are not strict medical terms defined in clinical anatomy, the area
below the lower eyelid, which was formed
with contraction of orbicularis oculi m., is
called the pretarsal roll with the lower line
below the pretarsal roll called the pretarsal
groove (Fig. 3.15).

Unlike Caucasians, the levator palpebral
superioris m. of Asians often do not attach to the
dermis. Relative to Caucasians, the orbital fat in
Asians extends further down, causing the eye to

Fig. 3.14 Sunken eye (**a**) and pretarsal roll (**b**) (Published with kind permission of © Hong-Ki Lee and Kwan-Hyun Youn 2016. All rights reserved)

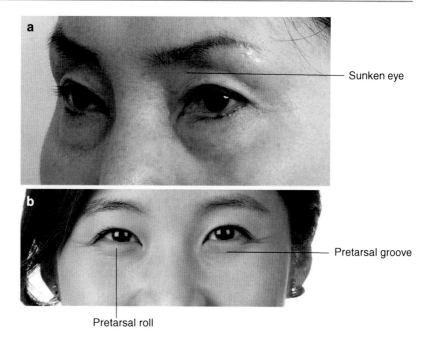

Sunken eye

Pretarsal groove

Pretarsal roll

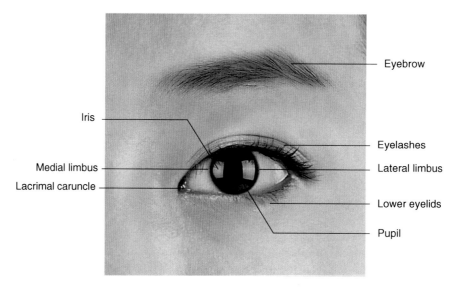

Eyebrow

Iris

Eyelashes

Medial limbus

Lateral limbus

Lacrimal caruncle

Lower eyelids

Pupil

Fig. 3.15 Basic nomenclature of the eye and periorbital region (Published with kind permission of © Kwan-Hyun Youn 2016. All rights reserved)

appear more swollen (Fig. 3.16). However, with aging, the orbital fat may decrease, leading to a pronounced orbital margin and to the appearance of a furrow below the eye which is also defined as a sunken eye. In this case, filler injections may alleviate the appearance of a sunken eye and reduce the symptoms of aging and fatigue.

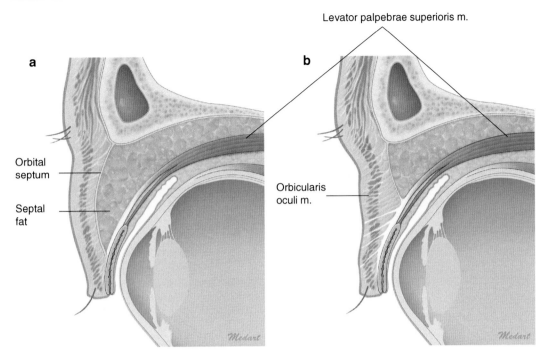

Fig. 3.16 Sagittal section of the upper eyelid and eyeball (**a** Asian, **b** Caucasian) (Published with kind permission of © Kwan-Hyun Youn 2016. All rights reserved)

3.2.2   Injection Points and Methods

Regarding treatment for a sunken eye, the patient's choice is most important. Filler injection may alleviate in case of a decrease of fat in the orbital roof in aged person. However, it is best that patients of the following types avoid filler injections as a possible for the treatment for sunken eyes. Firstly, if patients have ptosis, because of atrophy of muscles responsible for the movement of eyelids, increasing the volume of the upper eyelids by filler treatment may aggravate ptosis. Since sunken eyes may result from myasthenia gravis, a person's immunity and health condition should be checked before any treatment. Secondly, there is a limit to filler injections in treating sunken eyes, which result from exophthalmos.

Since the use of firm fillers may result in undulations when the patient closes his or her eyes, the use of soft fillers is recommended for treating sunken eyes. Therefore, it is important that filler injection occur only after taking into consideration on volume changes of a patient's upper eyelids in their opened and closed states.

Since it is both difficult and dangerous to inject fillers into the septal fat inside the orbital septum, injection points should be placed at the level of the orbital septum. Furthermore, soft fillers can be used to inject into the subcutaneous fat. A cannula is advised to avoid intra-arterial injection and should be inserted to the point slightly touching the periosteum and then slightly withdrawn so that it is placed in the orbital septum. If the cannula fails to penetrate a sufficient depth, undulations may appear when the eye is closed (Figs. 3.17 and 3.18).

The recommended forms of anesthesia during pretarsal roll treatment are infraorbital nerve block or specialized anesthetic ointment. Too deep injection during pretarsal roll treatment will result in a faulty shape, while too shallow injection will result in the filler showing through the surface of the skin; therefore, it is advised that the

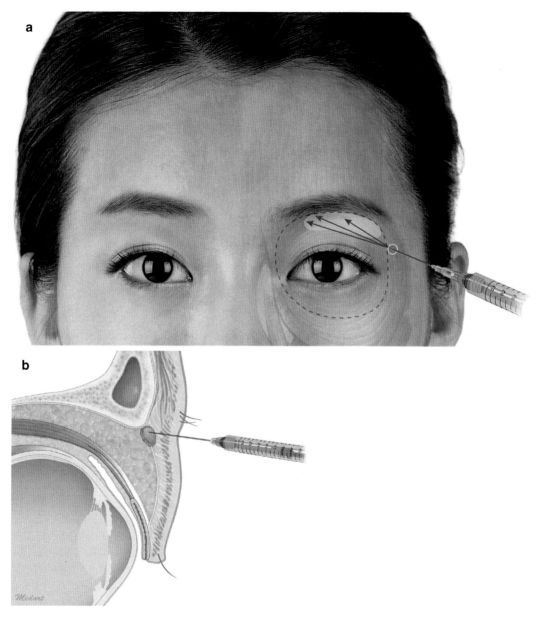

Fig. 3.17 Filler injection technique for sunken eye using cannula (**a**) and ideal injection plane (**b**) (Published with kind permission of © Hee-Jin Kim and Kwan-Hyun Youn 2016. All rights reserved)

injection take place at the subcutaneous tissue layer. In order to prevent the risk of excessive protrusion and sinking of the pretarsal roll, it is advised that the cannula or needle be inserted while keeping a minimum distance with the lower eyelash (Figs. 3.19 and 3.20). At the pretarsal roll, the inferior medial palpebral artery, a branch of the ophthalmic artery, locates in every case (Fig. 3.20a). This arterial branch supplies the tarsal plate of the lower eyelids, and its diameter is about 1 mm at the medial canthus. In this reason, too deep filler injection near the tarsal plate using a needle may cause the direct intravascular injection through the ophthalmic artery (Fig. 3.20b).

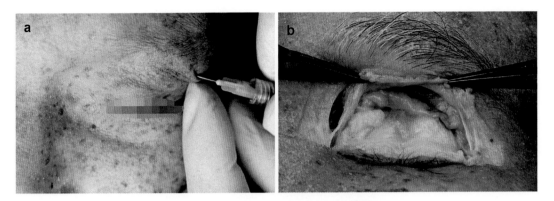

Fig. 3.18 Filler injection on the cadaveric sunken eye (**a**) and the properly located filler products (*green*) beneath the orbital septum and below orbital roof (**b**) (Published with kind permission of © Hee-Jin Kim 2016. All rights reserved)

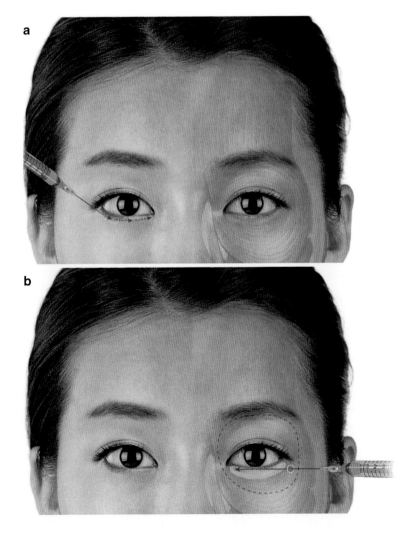

Fig. 3.19 Filler injection techniques for the pretarsal roll using needle (**a**) and cannula (**b**) (Published with kind permission of © Kwan-Hyun Youn 2016. All rights reserved)

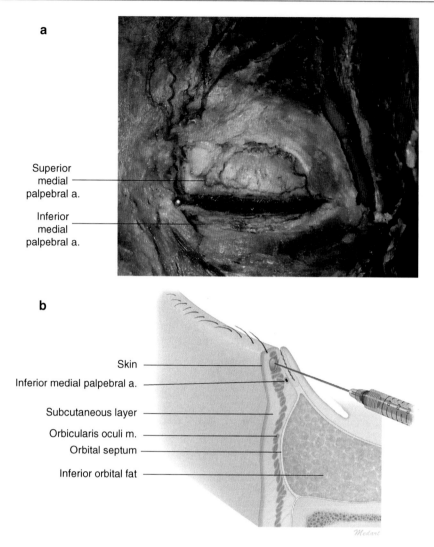

Fig. 3.20 Superior and inferior medial palpebral arteries distributing to the upper and lower eyelids from the ophthalmic artery (**a**) and filler injection plane for pretarsal roll using needle or cannula (**b**) (Published with kind permission of © Hee-Jin Kim 2016. All rights reserved)

The desired shape and volume of the pretarsal roll should be determined after observing the patient's smiling face. The general goal of the treatment should be to allow the pretarsal roll to become slightly more pronounced even when the patient is not smiling. Since the pretarsal roll can be formed with various shapes, such as becoming wider from the lateral 1/3 area or becoming more apparent at the lateral end, the filler injection must focus on accommodating the natural shape of the patient's pretarsal roll (Fig. 3.21).

Before injecting the pretarsal roll, the amount of inferior orbital fat present (inferior fat bulging) must be confirmed. Some patients possess an excess of inferior orbital fat, which pushes down on the pretarsal roll. In this case, proper surgical removal of some inferior orbital fat may allow the pretarsal roll to become eminent. In other cases, the pretarsal roll may only become visible when the patient smiles since the inferior orbital fat combines with the pretarsal roll to allow it to become more pronounced. In this case, the injec-

Resting state **Smiling state**

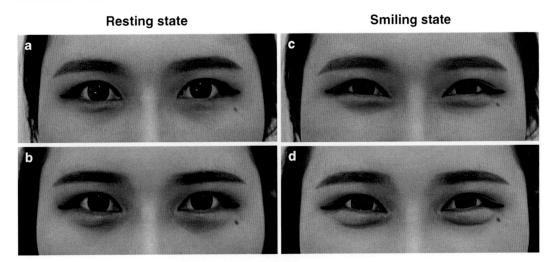

Fig. 3.21 Pretarsal roll injection using filler before (**a**, **c**) and after (**b**, **d**) injection (Published with kind permission of © Jisoo Kim 2016. All rights reserved)

tors consider the possibility of the pretarsal roll treatment resulting in an excessive protrusion of the pretarsal roll upon smiling. The success of this treatment relies heavily on the injector's ability to control the amount of filler after taking into consideration the elasticity of a patient's pretarsal groove. Inferior stretching of the pretarsal groove can be prevented by applying pressure on the lower area of the pretarsal groove by a finger or cotton swab while injecting the filler in small amounts.

It is highly recommended that soft fillers with low hydrophilic properties be used. The use of relatively rigid fillers will result in the pretarsal roll appearing uneven and lumpy. However, hydrophilic fillers will result in the pretarsal roll possessing an excessive volume. The optimal method of pretarsal roll treatment is to inject the sufficient soft filler and to make proper shape. In order to prevent any unnatural lumps and discontinued point could be corrected by putting cotton swab instantly after injection.

Since pretarsal roll treatment via filler injection targets the subdermal or intramuscular layers, the effects of filler treatment last longer than other filler treatments in other areas. Effect could last over three years with proper injection.

Bruising, resulting from the use of a needle during pretarsal roll treatment, may cause the patient discomfort. Therefore, the use of a 30–33 G-sized needle is advised. Furthermore, caution must be applied to avoid arteries that run close to the skin.

3.2.3 Side Effects

At the medial aspect of the septal fat, emergence of ophthalmic arterial branches, vessels may be thick (Fig. 3.22). Since this emergence point marks the beginning of many important arteries that run throughout the face, forehead, and nose and eventually communicates deeper with the central retinal a., a special attention is strongly advised when injecting into this area.

3.3 Temple

A depressed temple may give off an elderly and tired look (Fig. 3.23). Injection of fillers into the temple area can lead to a smoother line from the side of the forehead to the zygomatic prominence.

Fig. 3.22 Blood supply on the upper and lower lid from the ophthalmic artery (Published with kind permission of © Hee-Jin Kim 2016. All rights reserved)

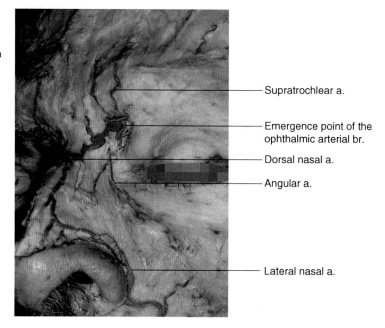

Supratrochlear a.

Emergence point of the ophthalmic arterial br.

Dorsal nasal a.

Angular a.

Lateral nasal a.

Fig. 3.23 Temple depression. It can be seen better when lowering one's head and looking above (Published with kind permission of © Jisoo Kim 2016. All rights reserved)

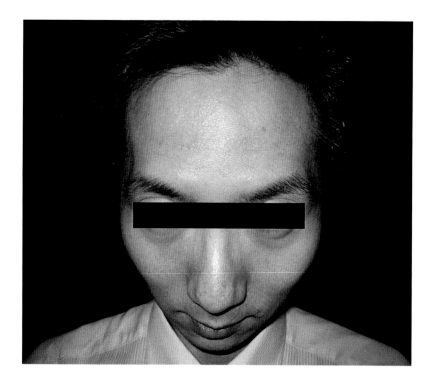

3.3.1 Clinical Anatomy

From a dictionary definition, the temporal region refers to the hollow region on the side of the head containing the temporal fossa. On the other hand, the temple refers to a smaller area around the pterion and is actually located slightly in front of the pterion from clinical perspectives. The temporalis m. occupies the temporal fossa with two distinct fascial layers on this muscle. The temporoparietal fascia (TPF), or the superficial temporal fascia, is a fascia located deep to the skin covering the temple region and surrounds the superficial temporal a. and v., which continue below as SMAS (Fig. 3.24).

Deep to the superficial temporal fascia, the deep temporal fascia or the temporalis muscle fascia covering the temporalis muscle is located. The superficial layer of the temporalis m. originated from this fascia. The deep temporal fascia attaches to the superior temporal line and traverses below to diverge into two layers (superficial and deep layers of the deep temporal fascia) that attach to the zygomatic arch. The space that forms as the deep temporal fascia splits into superficial and deep layers consists of a slight amount of fat tissue and the middle temporal vein (Fig. 3.25).

The middle temporal v. runs about 20 mm above the zygomatic arch, and this distance is approximately the width of the index finger when placed at the upper margin of the zygomatic arch. It is pivotal that the injector becomes familiar with the relative location of the middle temporal v. prior to filler treatment. The sentinel v., the inferior palpebral v., and the periorbital v. drain into the middle temporal v., which continues to the superficial temporal v., and flow further into the venous system of the neck (Figs. 3.25 and 3.26).

The deep temporal a. from the maxillary a. branches into the temporalis m., located in the deep temporal fascia. This artery gives branches into the anterior and posterior deep temporal a. between the temporal bone and the temporalis muscle. It then traverses upward to the temporal fossa, branching at the temporalis m. and fascia. The vascular layer is located below the belly and the tendon of the lower portion of the temporalis muscle. However, as the vessels traverse to the upper portion of the temporalis m., the vessels distribute throughout the muscle (Fig. 3.27).

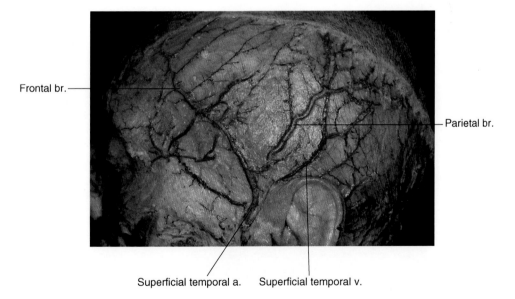

Frontal br.

Parietal br.

Superficial temporal a.   Superficial temporal v.

Fig. 3.24 Superficial temporal artery and vein enclosed within the temporoparietal fascia (Published with kind permission of © Hee-Jin Kim 2016. All rights reserved)

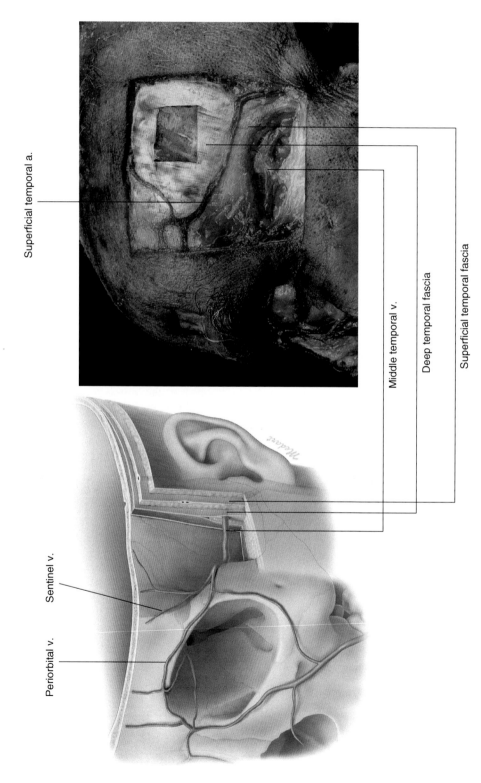

Superficial temporal a.

Middle temporal v.

Deep temporal fascia

Superficial temporal fascia

Sentinel v.

Periorbital v.

Fig. 3.25 Anatomical layers of the temple (Published with kind permission of © Hee-Jin Kim and Kwan-Hyun Youn 2016. All rights reserved)

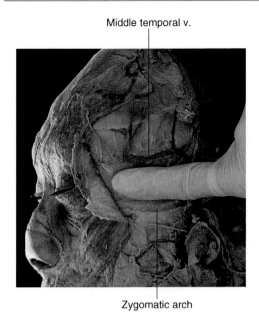

Middle temporal v.

Zygomatic arch

Fig. 3.26 Middle temporal vein (Published with kind permission of © Hee-Jin Kim 2016. All rights reserved)

3.3.2 Injection Points and Methods

In case of the filler injection using cannula, the anesthesia is needed. However, it is difficult to anesthetize this area. A zygomaticotemporal nerve block can be attempted, but it is most likely that the anesthesia will be ineffective. In order to reduce possible pain, it is highly advised to use lidocaine-contained fillers. When injecting with a needle, lidocaine-contained fillers is often sufficient for anesthesia. The use of a needle is advised when there is a focal depression in the temporal region; the use of a cannula is advised for a diffused area. The temporal region contains many blood vessels, and there have been reported cases of blindness caused by faulty filler injections. Although the exact cause is unknown, caution is advised to avoid intravascular injection.

When injecting into the depressed temple region, the filler should be injected at the depth

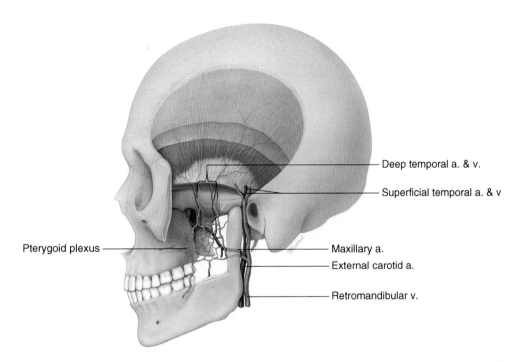

Deep temporal a. & v.

Superficial temporal a. & v

Pterygoid plexus

Maxillary a.

External carotid a.

Retromandibular v.

Fig. 3.27 Distribution of the deep temporal artery and vein within temporalis muscle (Published with kind permission of © Kwan-Hyun Youn 2016. All rights reserved)

of the periosteum. In this case, the injection should take place between the temporal fossa and the temporalis muscle. Because the depressed temple area is so large, it is cumbersome to treat even with a relatively large amount of fillers (Figs. 3.28a, 3.29, and 3.31).

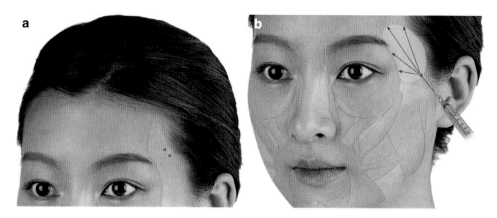

Fig. 3.28 Filler injection techniques for temple depression using needle (**a**) and cannula (**b**) (Published with kind permission of © Kwan-Hyun Youn 2016. All rights reserved)

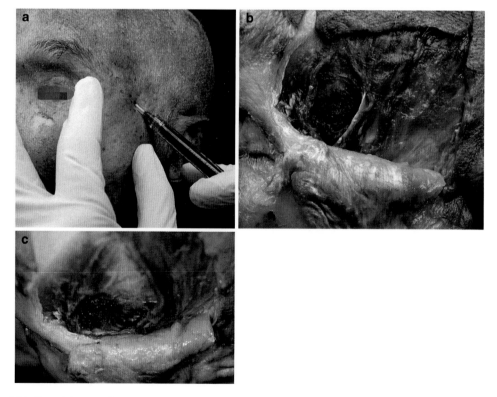

Fig. 3.29 Deep injection of filler on the cadaveric temple depression (**a**) and the dissection of the specimen to show the location of the filler product beneath the temporalis muscle (**b**, **c**) (Published with kind permission of © Hee-Jin Kim 2016. All rights reserved)

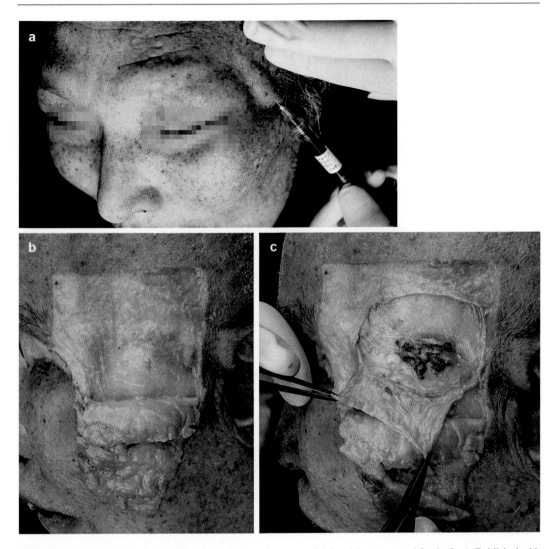

Fig. 3.30 Superficial injection of filler on the cadaveric temple depression (**a**) and the dissection of the specimen to show the location of the filler product between the superficial and deep temporal fascia (**b, c**) (Published with kind permission of © Hee-Jin Kim 2016. All rights reserved)

Pinching the temporal area causes the temporoparietal fascia to stick to the skin and the deep temporal fascia to stick to the muscle-forming space between the two fasciae. This area has relatively low blood vessel presence; therefore, piercing this area with a cannula is relatively safe. When using a cannula, approaching near the zygomatic arch is safer than approaching near the frontal branch of the superficial temporal artery (Figs. 3.28b, 3.30, and 3.31).

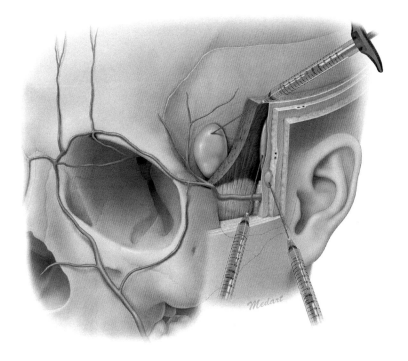

3.3.3 Side Effects

The pulse of the superficial temporal a. can easily be felt in front of the auricle. When injecting fillers into this area, it is advised that the path of the superficial temporal a. be considered by feeling its pulse. When injecting vertically into this area using a needle, caution is needed since the needle passes through multiple layers and can potentially damage blood vessels and even temporal bone. A lookout for hematoma is a good precautionary measure. Even though the use of a cannula is safer than a needle, it is recommended that the injection take place in an area with little to no vessels.

The locations of the sentinel v. and the middle temporal v. must be considered and avoided prior to the injection. Especially middle temporal v. runs parallel to the zygomatic arch passing between the superficial and deep layers of the deep temporal fascia. The middle temporal v. locates about 20 mm (one finger width) above the zygomatic arch. When an excess of fillers is injected, the zygomaticotemporal n. can be compressed with the elevation of local pressure despite unapparent symptoms.

Tip: Temple Filler Treatment The temple is the region easy to pass over during facial aesthetic procedure. The necessity and effective of filler injections in the temple may not be apparent, especially among females, since the temple is often covered by hair.

Filler injections in the temple should be performed after evaluating the patient's entire face. For a person with a generally lean face, filler injection into the temple may not result in patient satisfaction. On the other hand, a patient with the depressed temple with prominent zygomatic arch is more likely to feel highly satisfied after filler injection into the temple region. Furthermore, a physician must accurately pinpoint which areas in the temple are depressed. Most importantly, filler injection should be carried out to create a smooth contour between the forehead and the zygoma.

Tip: Four Possible Layers of Filler Injection into the Temple There are generally four possible layers of injection when treating the temple. The first layer is the area between the temporoparietal fascia (superficial temporal fascia) and the deep temporal fascia; the second layer is the area between the superficial and the deep layer of the deep temporal fascia; the third is the area between the deep temporal fascia and temporalis muscle; and the fourth layer is the area between the temporalis m. and the bone of the temporal fossa.

When injecting into the first layer between the temporoparietal fascia and the deep temporal fascia, the use of a cannula is advised to minimize the possibility of damaging the superficial temporal a. and v. and the frontal branch of the facial nerve. Intravascular injection into the superficial temporal a. must be avoided since it is the main artery that supplies blood to the upper and lateral forehead. Massaging the area of injection is pivotal since undulations may appear due to the thin skin in the temple region. In order to minimize bruising and vessel damage, the cannula should be placed targeting the layer above the deep temporal fascia.

The superficial temporal fat pad and the middle temporal v. are present in the second layer between the superficial and the deep layer of the deep temporal fascia. A branch of the middle temporal v. converges with the sentinel v., the inferior palpebral v., and the periorbital v. to drain into the superficial temporal v. and enter the venous system of the neck. If intravascular injections of fillers were to occur, a sudden increase in intravascular pressure would lead to a back flow of blood and filler into the cavernous sinus via the periorbital v. and the superior ophthalmic vein. Therefore, when injecting into the second layer, the location of the middle temporal v., 2 cm above the zygomatic arch must be confirmed. An

aspiration prior to the injection is strongly advised to avoid the intravascular injection.

The space between deep temporal fascia and temporalis muscle is potential space where can be created with proper placement of needle and cannula just deep to the deep temporal fascia. The injection on this layer is usually carried out with cannula after piercing deep temporal fascial. This layer is relative avascular space superficial to the temporalis muscle. After making entry point with needle until temporalis muscle layer, cannula should be inserted into the superficial temporal fascia and deep temporal fascia. Just after placing the tip of cannula below the deep temporal fascia, the cannula should be directed parallel to the muscle plane. After instillation, adequate amount of filler, the manual compression of massage should be applied to even the surface.

Injections into the fourth layer over the bone surface of the temporal fossa are relatively safe, because the deep temporal arteries. and vv. tend to only provide blood to muscles, while direct communications with other vessels are few. Nevertheless, in order to avoid injecting the filler directly into the blood vessel, the bone surface of the temporal fossa should first be checked with the needle. A safer injection can be made into the bone surface deep to the muscle by using the bevel-down technique, after touching the bone with needle tip, in which an injection is superiorly and inferiorly made obliquely at a 45° angle. In this area, the blood vessel locates within the muscle rather than at the bone surface of the temporal fossa. Therefore, risks to the blood vessel can be reduced if the bevel is made to approach to the bone surface. In order to approach the bone surface of the temporal fossa, using a needle of sufficient length is recommended. When injecting into the fourth layer, it is safer and holds the advantage of having fewer possibilities of experiencing irregularities on the surface. However, the injection should be performed taking into account the disadvantage of a possibly needing a greater volume of filler due to the tension from a tight deep temporal fascia.

Suggested Reading

Muscles of the Face and Neck

1. Lee JY, Kim JN, Kim SH, Choi HG, Hu KS, Kim HJ,
Song WC, Koh KS. Anatomical verification and designation of the superficial layer of the temporalis
muscle. Clin Anat. 2012;25(2):176–81.

Vessels of the Face and Neck

2. Jung W, Youn KH, Won SY, Park JT, Hu KS, Kim
HJ. Clinical implications of the middle temporal vein
with regard to temporal fossa augmentation. Dermatol
Surg. 2014;40(6):618–23.
3. Lee HJ, Kang IW, Won SY, Lee JG, Hu KS, Tansatit
T, Kim HJ. Description of a novel anatomical venous
structure in the nasoglabellar area. J Craniofac Surg.
2014;25(2):633–5.

4. Lee JG, Yang HM, Hu KS, Lee YI, Lee HJ, Choi YJ,
Kim HJ. Frontal branch of the superficial temporal
artery: anatomical study and clinical implications
regarding injectable treatments. Surg Radiol Anat.
2015;37(1):61–8.
5. Yang HM, Jung W, Won SY, Youn KH, Hu KS,
Kim HJ. Anatomical study of medial zygomaticotemporal vein and its clinical implication regarding the injectable treatments. Surg Radiol Anat.
2014;37(2):175–80.

Peripheral Nerves of the Face and Neck

6. Won SY, Kim DH, Yang HM, Park JT, Kwak HH, Hu
KS, Kim HJ. Clinical and anatomical approach using
Sihler's staining technique (whole mount nerve stain).
Anat Cell Biol. 2011;44(1):1–7.

Clinical Anatomy of the Midface for Filler Injection

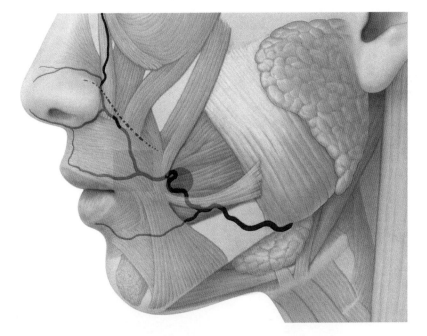

Kyle K. Seo, MD, PhD & Hee-Jin Kim, DDS, PhD (Illustrated by Dr. Kwan-Hyun Youn)

© Springer Science+Business Media Singapore 2016
H.-J. Kim et al., *Clinical Anatomy of the Face for Filler and Botulinum Toxin Injection*,
DOI 10.1007/978-981-10-0240-3_4

4.1   Tear Trough

4.1.1   Clinical Anatomy

Tear troughs are dented regions of the periorbital hollow located 1/3 medially below the eye. The lower eyelid can create a shadow in this area, which results in a tired look (Fig. 4.1).

Tear troughs form at the border where relatively thin skin from the eyebrow meets relatively thick skin from the nose. Tear troughs may appear in people of all ages. The pronunciations of tear troughs occur for various reasons; nonetheless, the reduction of volume in tissues surrounding the periorbital region is the most significant reason.

Orbital fat herniation, stretching of the skin, and volume changes in tissues can serve as additional causes. Dissecting a cadaver reveals two to three orbicularis retaining ligaments (ORL) pinching the orbicularis oculi muscle deep to the bone. In actuality, the sagging periorbital region joins the inferior muscle fibers of the orbicularis oculi m. to create the image of being suspended by the ORL

fibers. In addition, the projected angle of the sagging fat inferior to the periorbital region can be observed (Fig. 4.2).

The ORLs serve as an anchor from the orbicularis oculi m. to the orbit. The orbicularis oculi m. is directly attached to the bone from the anterior lacrimal crest to the medial orbital margin. The ORL replaces the muscle at this point to follow the orbit and extend laterally. The medial portion of the ORL is firmly attached to the deep portion of the orbicularis oculi muscle (Fig. 4.3a). On the other hand, the lateral portion of the ORL differs from its medial portion in that it consists of the loose and elongated septum (Fig. 4.3b).

It is certain that the ORLs that attach to the surface of the orbital margin consist of several—not single—ligaments that link further to the deep layer of the orbicularis oculi muscle. However, there are no direct attachments by ORL into the dermis of the skin (Fig. 4.4).

The inferior palpebral v. and angular v. traverse the area near the tear trough; therefore, the use of a cannula is advised in order to prevent bruising (Fig. 4.5).

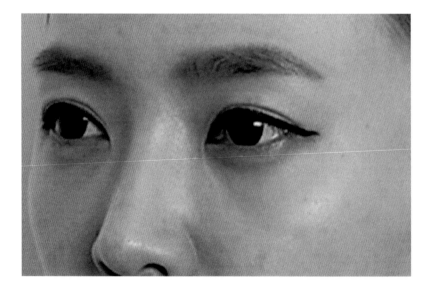

Fig. 4.1 Tear trough (Published with kind permission of © Kyle K Seo 2016. All rights reserved)

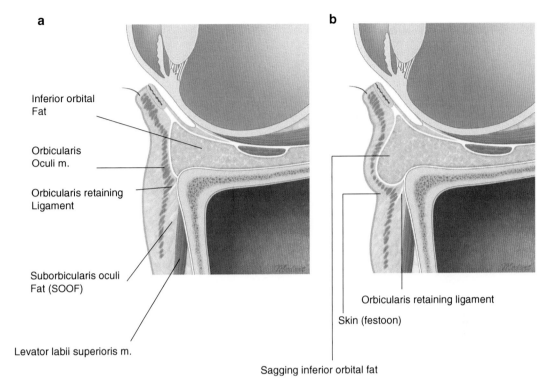

Fig. 4.2 Sagittal section of the lower eyelid in young (**a**) and aged person (**b**) (Published with kind permission of © Kwan-Hyun Youn 2016. All rights reserved)

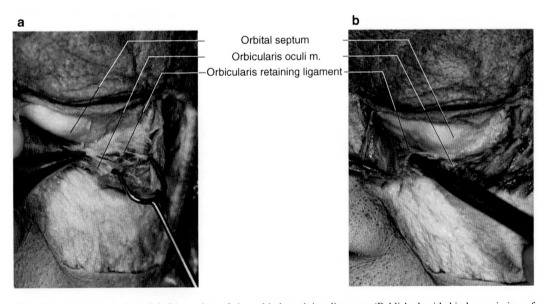

Fig. 4.3 Lateral (**a**) and medial (**b**) portion of the orbital retaining ligament (Published with kind permission of © Hee-Jin Kim 2016. All rights reserved)

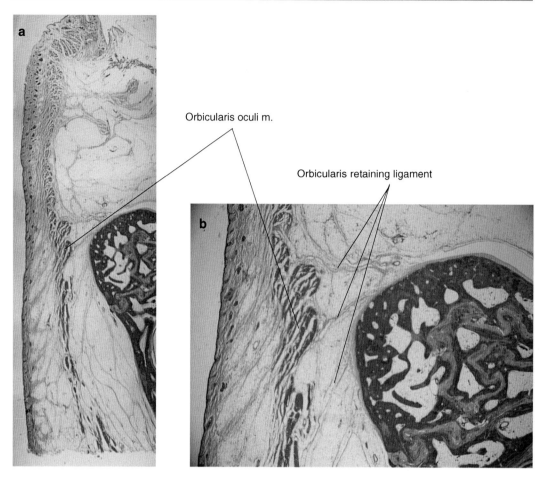

Orbicularis oculi m.

Orbicularis retaining ligament

Fig. 4.4 Histologic section of the lower eyelid having a normal contour of lid-cheek junction (**a**) and its magnified micrograph (**b**) (Published with kind permission of © Hee-Jin Kim 2016. All rights reserved)

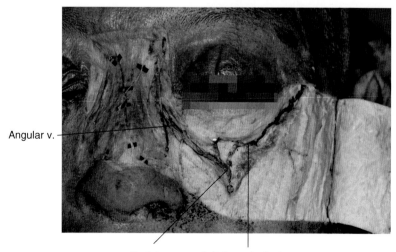

Angular v.

Facial v.   Inferior palpebral v.

Fig. 4.5 Inferior palpebral vein (Published with kind permission of © Hee-Jin Kim 2016. All rights reserved)

4.1.2 Injection Points and Methods

Filler injection should proceed with two layers in mind. When the atrophy of the soft tissue located below the ORL is severe, the filler should be injected deep into the suborbicularis oculi fat (SOOF) layer of the prezygomatic space in order to restore volume. When the volume of the SOOF is restored, the filler should be injected into the subcutaneous tissue located on the upper part of the orbicularis oculi m. to give a detailed finish (Figs. 4.6 and 4.22a). Normally, filler injection into the superficial layer of the orbicularis oculi m. results in lump of filler; however, filler treatment on the tear trough is an exception, with filler injection into the superficial layer of the orbicularis oculi m. resulting in better clinical outcomes.

Only HA fillers must be used. Since fillers containing collagen derivatives such as calcium may clump, these types of fillers should not be used on patients with thin skin. HA fillers with a low water retention capacity should be recommended, because HA fillers with a high water retention capacity may occur with persistent swelling 1–2 weeks after injection. Besides, sufficient soft filler with very low viscoelasticity should be recommended to prevent lump.

Since many blood vessels traverse the orbital region, the use of a cannula is strongly advised. The entry point of the cannula should be in a straight line 1 cm away from the end of the tear trough (Fig. 4.7). When injecting into the SOOF layer, a cannula of size 23–27 G is advised; when injecting into the superficial layer of the orbicularis oculi m., the use of a 30 G cannula is recommended.

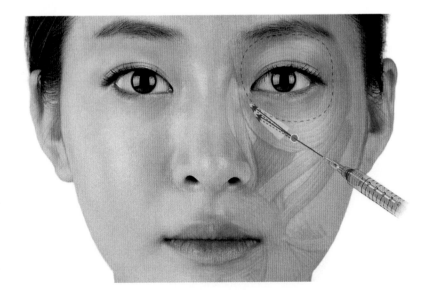

Fig. 4.6 Filler injection techniques on the tear trough using cannula (Published with kind permission of © Kwan-Hyun Youn 2016. All rights reserved)

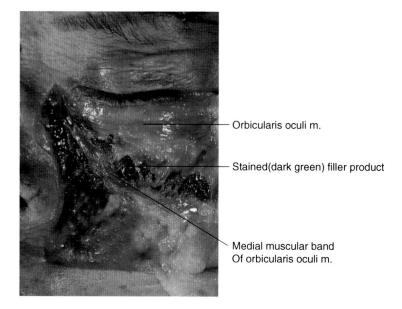

Fig. 4.7 Properly injected filler in the SOOF for the treatment of tear trough of the cadaveric specimen (green-tinged filler product) (Published with kind permission of © Hee-Jin Kim 2016. All rights reserved)

Orbicularis oculi m.

Stained(dark green) filler product

Medial muscular band Of orbicularis oculi m.

4.2　Nasojugal Groove

4.2.1　Clinical Anatomy

The nasojugal groove refers to a drooping of the area extending from the medial canthus to the anterior zygomatic region. The nasojugal groove may include the tear trough (Fig. 4.8). Regardless of ages, the nasojugal groove could extend into the midcheek furrow (Indian band). The depression of the lower orbital region not only leads to a pronounced dark circles but also leads to a tired, elderly look.

The anterior zygomatic region consists of the following tissue layers: skin, superficial layer of malar fat, orbicularis oculi m., suborbicularis oculi fat (SOOF), muscle layer of levator labii superioris m. and zygomaticus minor m., and periosteum of the maxilla where the infraorbital nn. emerge (Fig. 4.9). In this region, zygomatic cutaneous ligaments locate along the lower margin of the orbicularis oculi muscle (Fig. 4.10).

The orbicularis oculi m. serves to separate the malar fat pad into superficial and deep layers. The portion of the deep layer located below the orbicularis oculi m. is called as the suborbicularis oculi fat (SOOF) (Fig. 4.11). The distribution of fat composing the malar fat pad changes with age. Aging not only results in the attenuation and drooping of the lower portion of the SOOF but also results in the sagging of the malar fat pad

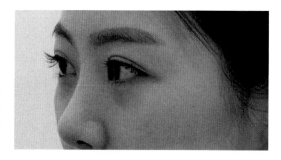

Fig. 4.8 Nasojugal groove (Published with kind permission of © Jisoo Kim 2016. All rights reserved)

above the nasolabial fold. On the other hand, the zygomatic cutaneous ligament supports and prevents drooping of the upper portion of the SOOF, so the malar fat pad can be divided into an upper and lower portion by the nasojugal groove. If protrusion of the inferior orbital fat is accompanied by ptosis of the lower eyelid, the sagging of the tear troughs becomes intensified.

In about 30% of Asians, angular arteries detour around the anterior zygomatic region while following the inferomedial border of the medial muscular band of orbicularis oculi muscle. Therefore, when injecting fillers into the nasojugal groove, caution must be taken to avoid damaging this artery (Fig. 4.12). The use of a cannula is strongly suggested. Even using cannula, caution must be taken not to pierce facial blood vessels with excessive pressure.

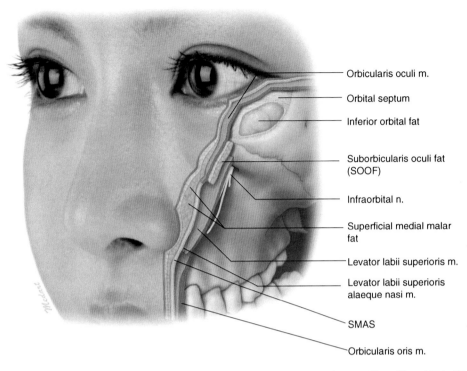

Orbicularis oculi m.

Orbital septum

Inferior orbital fat

Suborbicularis oculi fat (SOOF)

Infraorbital n.

Superficial medial malar fat

Levator labii superioris m.

Levator labii superioris alaeque nasi m.

SMAS

Orbicularis oris m.

Fig. 4.9 Anatomical layers of the midface (Published with kind permission of © Kwan-Hyun Youn 2016. All rights reserved)

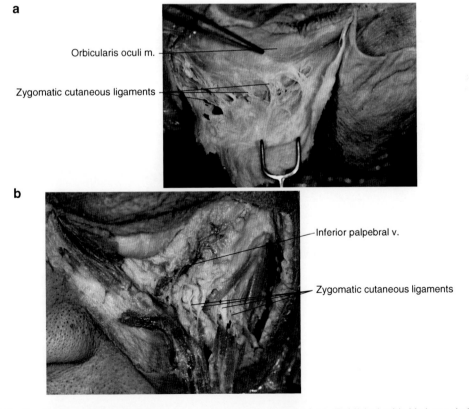

a

Orbicularis oculi m.

Zygomatic cutaneous ligaments

b

Inferior palpebral v.

Zygomatic cutaneous ligaments

Fig. 4.10 Zygomatic cutaneous ligaments (**a** superior view, **b** frontal view) (Published with kind permission of © Hee-Jin Kim 2016. All rights reserved)

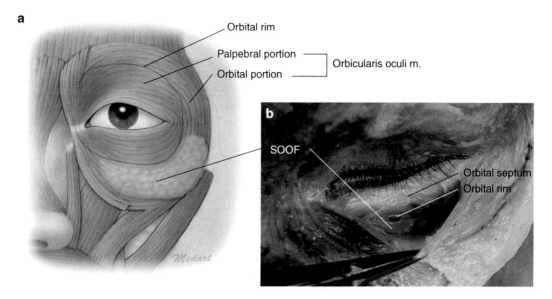

Fig. 4.11 Anatomy of the suborbicularis oculi fat (*SOOF*). (**a**) Dissection of the lower eyelid revealing the upper portion of suborbicularis oculi fat (SOOF) (**b** supe-rior view) (Published with kind permission of © Kwan-Hyun Youn 2016. All rights reserved)

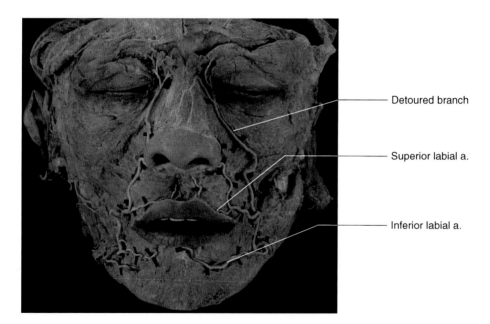

Fig. 4.12 Detoured branch of the facial artery along the nasojugal groove (Published with kind permission of © Hee-Jin Kim 2016. All rights reserved)

4.2.2 Injection Points and Methods

Filler injection depth should be the level of the prezygomatic space deep to SOOF layer (Figs. 4.13a and 4.22). Although it is generally mentioned that the injection should target just above the periosteum within the prezygomatic space, the injections specifically target the deeper SOOF layer above the levator labii superioris and the zygomaticus minor muscle. Firstly, fillers should be injected deep into the SOOF layer to fill the sunken portions of the prezygomatic space. Secondly, fillers should be injected into the subcutaneous layer above the orbicularis oculi muscle.

The filler injection should take place according to principle with the filler first being injected at the central portion of the most sunken area and the rest of the filler being injected accordingly above and below the central portion to create a natural curvature.

The use of a cannula is recommended due to the abundant blood vessels in this region. Normally, the point of cannula insertion should be placed vertically at a 1 cm distance from the lower end of the nasojugal groove. In most cases, the injection entry point corresponds to the point where the perpendicular line starting from lateral canthus intersects with the horizontal line passing the inferior border of nasal ala (Fig. 4.13b, c). However, the injection entry point should be adjusted according to the length and direction of the nasojugal groove. When injecting into the SOOF layer for the purpose of volume restoration, use of a HA filler in combination with a 23–27 G cannula is advised. Cannula size is decided depending on filler product. Instead of the filler containing calcium

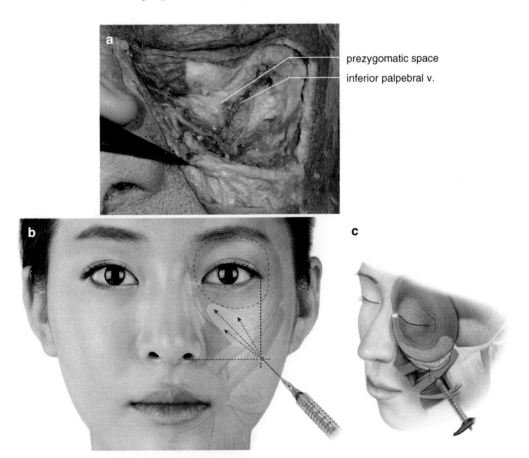

prezygomatic space
inferior palpebral v.

Fig. 4.13 The prezygomatic space under the orbicularis oculi muscle (**a**) and filler injection techniques for and nasojugal groove using cannula (**b**, **c**) (Published with kind permission of © Hee-Jin Kim 2016. All rights reserved)

and collagen derivatives, HA filler that can be dissolved is the safest.

4.3 Palpebromalar Groove

4.3.1 Clinical Anatomy

The palpebromalar groove forms along the lower lateral orbital rim between the lateral aspect of the lower eyelid and the zygoma. The palpebromalar groove may be uneven and lumpy, leading to a pronunciation of dark circles. The palpebromalar groove can be formed by protrusion of inferior orbital fat and accumulation of the malar mound fat pad (Fig. 4.14).

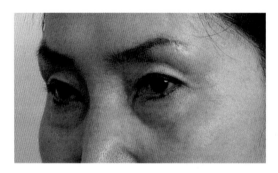

Fig. 4.14 Palpebromalar groove (Published with kind permission of © Kyle K Seo 2016. All rights reserved)

4.3.2 Injection Points and Methods

The cannula insertion point should be placed 0.5 cm apart from the lateral canthus (Fig. 4.15). A 30 G cannula should be used to fill the groove. First, the filler should be injected deeply into the internal aspect of the orbital septum to create a general increase in volume. If the volume generated is insufficient after deep injection, the filler should be injected slightly above the orbicularis oculi muscle.

4.4 Nasolabial Fold

4.4.1 Clinical Anatomy

The nasolabial fold begins at the alar groove and alar facial crease and runs down the lateral aspects of the upper lip. The nasolabial fold is not a simple crease, but is a unique three-dimensional curvature in that it is the result of a crease that forms as the medial boundary of the malar fat pad due to the cutaneous insertion of the upper lip elevators and the zygomaticus major muscle along nasolabial line. As a result, the nasolabial fold can be defined more as one of natural components of the face rather than a wrinkle that forms as a result of aging (Fig. 4.16).

Upper lip elevators, such as levator labii superioris alaeque nasi (LLSAN), levator labii superioris

Fig. 4.15 Filler injection techniques for the palpebromalar groove using cannula (Published with kind permission of © Kwan-Hyun Youn 2016. All rights reserved)

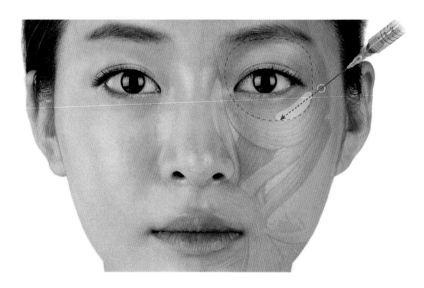

(LLS), and the zygomaticus minor (Zmi), attach to the skin at the nasolabial fold along their path to the upper lip and the orbicularis oris muscle (Fig. 4.17).

The nasolabial fold can become more pronounced deep and long due to sagging of the skin and the malar fat pad, atrophy of deep medial cheek fat, and changes in fat composition (Fig. 4.16). However, the attachment of upper lip elevator muscles to the skin on nasolabial fold makes malar fat not to descend further below nasolabial fold, but worsens a natural nasolabial fold. Besides, repeated muscle movement with age can create fine nasolabial wrinkles on skin.

In about 77 % of Asians, facial arteries traverse slightly toward the medial aspect of the

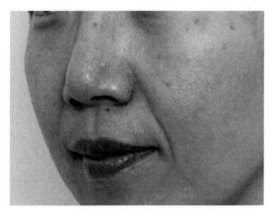

Fig. 4.16 Nasolabial fold (Published with kind permission of © Kyle K Seo 2016. All rights reserved)

nasolabial fold (Fig. 4.18); therefore, caution is advised to avoid risk of intravascular injection when injecting filler into this region. Furthermore, in about 56 % (nasolabial pattern (37 %) and forehead pattern (18.6 %), Fig. 1.43) of Asians, a part of the superior labial and the lateral nasal a. are exposed over the orbicularis oris m. at the medial aspect of the nasolabial fold. Caution should be taken when injecting superficially below the nasolabial fold as severe bruising may occur.

Facial Arteries and Nasolabial Folds in Asians
In 93.3 % of Asians, the facial a. runs close to the nasolabial fold. Figure 4.19 depicts the facial a. in relation to the nasolabial fold. The facial artery is located 3.2 ± 4.5 mm lateral from the nasal ala; the artery is also located 13.5 ± 5.4 mm apart from the cheilion.

In 42.9 % of Asians, the nasal division of the facial a. traverses the medial aspect of the nasolabial fold; in 23.2 % of Asians, the nasal division of the facial a. traverses the lateral aspect of nasolabial fold. In other cases (33.9 %), the facial a. crosses the nasolabial fold (Fig. 4.19). In 43 % of Asians, the facial a. ascended within 5 mm of the nasolabial fold.

In 30 % of Asians, the detoured branch of the facial a. (type II) runs along the nasojugal groove and turns medially over the infraorbital area (Fig. 4.20). The average distances are shown in Fig. 4.20.

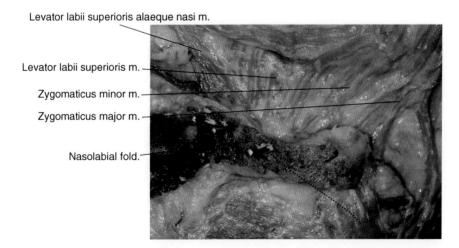

Levator labii superioris alaeque nasi m.
Levator labii superioris m.
Zygomaticus minor m.
Zygomaticus major m.
Nasolabial fold.

Fig. 4.17 Cutaneous insertion of parts of the upper lip elevators into the nasolabial fold (Published with kind permission of © Hee-Jin Kim 2016. All rights reserved)

Fig. 4.18 Facial arterial branch beneath the nasolabial fold (*dotted line*) (Published with kind permission of © Hee-Jin Kim 2016. All rights reserved)

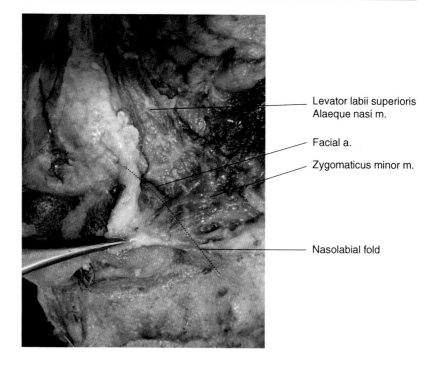

Levator labii superioris Alaeque nasi m.

Facial a.

Zygomaticus minor m.

Nasolabial fold

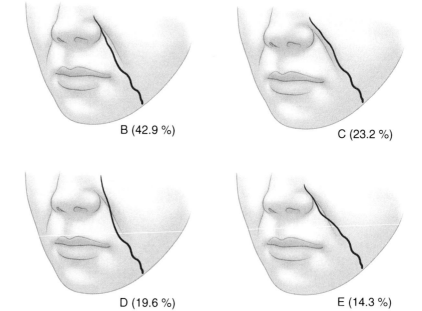

B (42.9 %)

C (23.2 %)

Fig. 4.19 Location of the facial artery with reference to the nasolabial fold in Korean and Thai population (Published with kind permission of © Kwan-Hyun Youn 2016. All rights reserved)

D (19.6 %)

E (14.3 %)

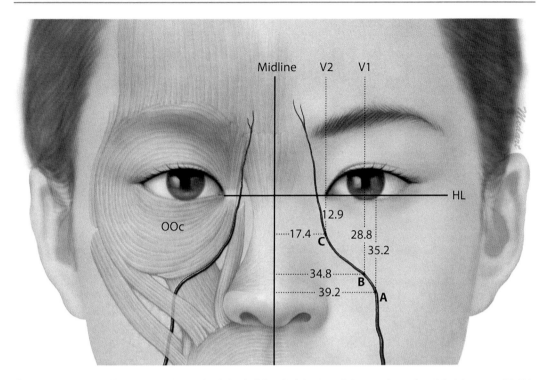

Fig. 4.20 Location of the detoured branch of the facial artery. *V1* vertical line through the midpoint between the medial and lateral canthus, *V2* vertical line through the medial canthus, *HL* horizontal line through medial canthi of both sides, *A* the turning point of the curvature of the facial artery, *B* the meeting point of facial artery with V1, *C* the meeting point of the facial artery with V2 (*OOc* orbicularis oculi m) (Published with kind permission of © Kwan-Hyun Youn 2016. All rights reserved)

4.4.2 Injection Points and Methods

Prior to injection for the nasolabial fold, a physician should imagine the nasolabial fold as an isosceles triangle. This triangle is composed of a baseline from the starting point of the alar groove to the inferior margin of the nasal ala, and the upper long side of triangle is the nasolabial fold. The other lower long side of the triangle is the concave sunken area below the nasolabial fold. Fillers should be injected with the objective of adjusting the volume of the lower sunken area of the isosceles triangle with the contour of the fat layer of the upper side of this triangle (Fig. 4.21).

First, volume restoration with filler should be performed within the canine fossa (Fig. 4.22); the filler should then be injected retrogradely

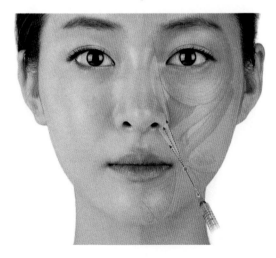

Fig. 4.21 Filler injection techniques for the nasolabial fold using cannula (Published with kind permission of © Kwan-Hyun Youn 2016. All rights reserved)

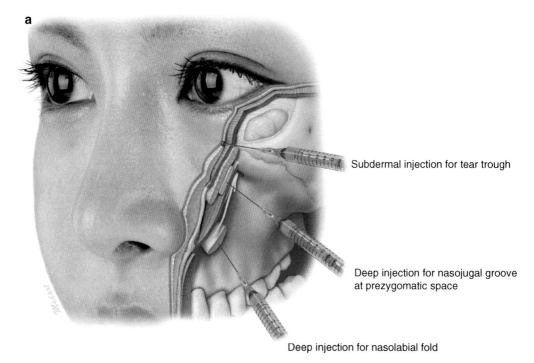

Subdermal injection for tear trough

Deep injection for nasojugal groove
at prezygomatic space

Deep injection for nasolabial fold

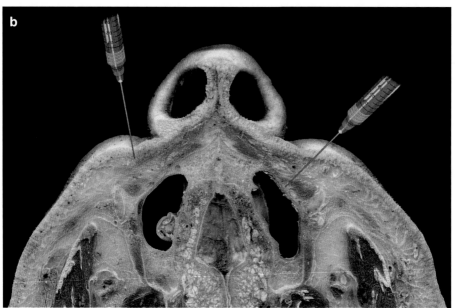

Fig. 4.22 Appropriate planes for filler injection on the midface (**a**) and two possible safe injection plane for nasolabial fold augmentation (**b**) (Published with kind permission of © Kwan-Hyun Youn 2016. All rights reserved)

from an injection point medially located 1–5 mm from the nasolabial fold. When injecting into the canine fossa, the injection should take place just above the periosteum. At the medial portion of the nasolabial fold, the injection takes place on the superficial layer of the

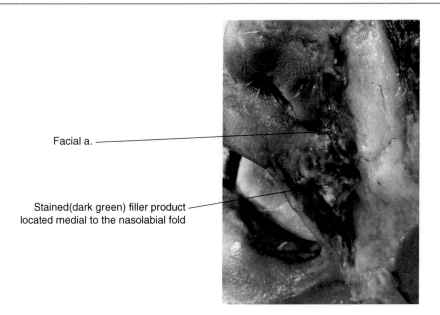

Facial a.

Stained(dark green) filler product
located medial to the nasolabial fold

Fig. 4.23 Cadaveric filler injection on the nasolabial fold using cannula (deep injection) (Published with kind permission of © Hee-Jin Kim 2016. All rights reserved)

orbicularis oris muscle (Fig. 4.23). Injecting into the dermis may also be an effective combination treatment when facial wrinkles are highly apparent (Fig. 4.22b).

Filler Treatment of the Nasolabial Fold and Facial Artery

Facial a. is the important point of caution. Ischemia of facial a. due to intravascular injection or extravascular compression can lead to necrosis of the skin. This is one of the most common side effects of filler injections. The facial a. is a cardinal facial vessel that arises from the external carotid artery. It is known to proceed superoanteriorly from the premasseteric area in front of the mandibular angle to the adjacent portion of the nasion. Facial a. gives branches of the inferior labial, the superior labial, the lateral nasal, and the angular a. on the face.

At the lower face, facial a. located deeper than the platysma and the depressor anguli oris muscle. As the artery traverses further upward, it runs between the risorius and the zygomaticus major m. immediately in front of the buccal fat pad. At this region, facial a. is not covered by any muscles. In this location, the facial a.

shows the appearance of a coiled snake or pig's tail; furthermore, the artery receives no protection from the muscle layer below the superficial fat layer. It is usually located lateral to the mouth corner (Fig. 4.24). Filler injections in this area can lead to rupturing of the facial a. followed by severe hematoma, bruising, and extensive edema. Hematoma should be taken into consideration if sudden external swelling on the cheek occurs or if patients express of the formation of acorn or chestnut during filler injection procedure.

In order to prevent the side effects stated above, a physician should constantly be aware of the presence of facial arterial branch beneath the facial skin during puncture with needle for entry; therefore, a physician should take care to make certain that the needle should penetrate the skin very slightly when forming the entry point for the cannula. Furthermore, a cannula of large size should be used—minimum size being 27 G—in order to lower the chance of piercing or damaging blood vessels. Moreover, the tip of the cannula should proceed first to the upper medial aspect near the side of the nose, and then retrograde slow injection of filler should be done after

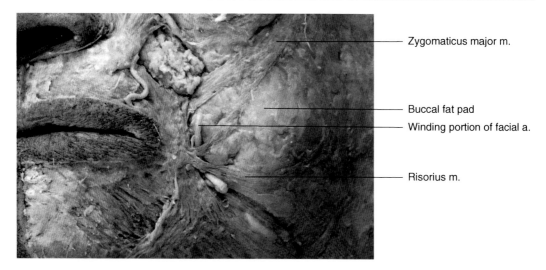

Fig. 4.24 Winding portion of the facial artery between risorius and zygomaticus major muscles without any muscle coverage (Published with kind permission of © Hee-Jin Kim 2016. All rights reserved)

Fig. 4.25 Two danger zones during filler injection for nasolabial fold (*green box* branching region of the superior labial artery, *purple circle* winding portion of the facial artery without any muscle coverage) (Published with kind permission of © Kwan-Hyun Youn 2016. All rights reserved)

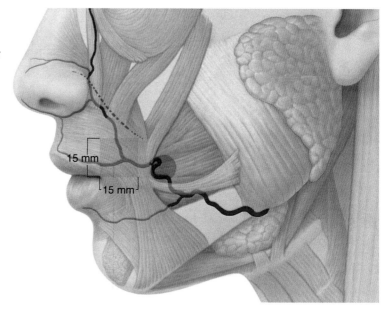

confirming the absence of the vascular damage. This procedure helps to prevent the filler from seeping into any damaged blood vessels.

The superolateral region from the mouth corner is another dangerous zone when injecting fillers into the nasolabial fold. The superior labial branch is the primary supplier of the upper lip. In most cases, the superior labial a. branches from the facial artery and its branching point is located at a 1.5-cm-side square superolateral to the cheilion (Fig. 4.25). After the superior labial artery

branched from facial artery, it ran superior to the vermilion border under the orbicularis oris muscle, with a minimum depth of 3 mm. It then courses inferior to the vermilion border before approaching the peak of Cupid's bow. Caution must be taken when injecting a needle into this area or when forming a cannula entry point with a needle. Therefore, when injecting fillers into the nasolabial fold, the insertion points should be made at a 1 cm apart from the ending of the naso-labial fold or a point of 1 cm lateral and 1 cm below, respectively, from the cheilion. The size of the cannula should vary within a range of 23–27 G according to the type of filler used (Fig. 4.22).

4.5   Hollow Cheek

4.5.1   Clinical Anatomy

The depression of the cheeks not only gives the appearance of aging and fatigue but also leads to a protrusion of the zygomatic arch. Among Asian populations that favor plump cheeks, filler treatment for hollow cheeks is relatively popular. Furthermore, depression of the anterior cheeks results in an accentuation of nasolabial folds by coinciding with the cheeks and the nasolabial folds (Fig. 4.26).

The cheek consists of the skin, subcutaneous fatty layer, facial mm. and SMAS, buccal fat pad, buccinators m., and oral mucosa (Fig. 4.27). Fat in the cheeks can be divided into a superficial layer of fat tissue above the facial m. and the buccal fat pad deep to the facial muscles. The buccal fat pad (Bichat's fat pad) is one of several encap-sulated fat tissues in the head. This fat pad is a deep fat pad located between the buccinators m. and several superficial muscles. The lower portion of the buccal fat pad is contained within the buccal space. The fat tissue consists of small lobules, and the two fat tissues can be distinguished even with the naked eye. The buccal fat pad is composed of the central body and extensions. The medial aspect of the central body (buccal lobe) is adjacent to the buccinators m.; the lateral aspect is surrounded by the masticatory m., some the facial mm., and the parotid gland (Figs. 4.27 and 4.28).

It should not be confused with the malar fat tissue located below the cheek skin. The extensions of the buccal fat pad are located at the pterygopalatine fossa (lobe), the temporal fossa (lobe), and the buccal space (lobe). From an aesthetic perspective, the central body and its extensions are extremely important in that they make up 50% of the total cheek fat and buccal fat atrophy with age aggravating the hollow cheek. The buccal fat pad is supported by the risorius m., and aging of the risorius m. often leads to sagging of the anterior cheek and to marionette lines (Fig. 4.28).

4.5.2   Insertion Points and Methods

The two possible layers of injection are the subcutaneous fat layer and the buccal fat pad (Fig. 4.29a). Since injecting into the buccal fat pad requires a large volume of filler even though hollow cheek is due to the atrophy of the buccal fat, filler injection into the buccal fat pad is not usually recommended except in cases of the severe sunken cheek. Due to the dense and compact nature of the buccal fat pad, filler injection may aggravate jowl sagging in some cases.

The ideal injection regions for the hollow cheek are the area from the nasolabial fold to the masseter m. and the area from the lower portion of the zygomatic arch to the sagging point of the cheek. In this case, the use of a cannula is also recommended because of the wide target area. The entry of the cannula should be placed 1 cm lateral to and 2 cm below the mouth corner (cheilion) (Fig. 4.29b). Although the collagen derivatives such as a calcium filler can be used, the use of a degradable HA filler is highly advised.

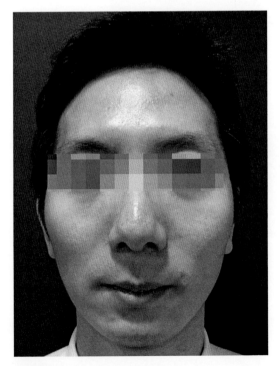

Fig. 4.26 Hollow cheek (Published with kind permission of © Jisoo Kim 2016. All rights reserved)

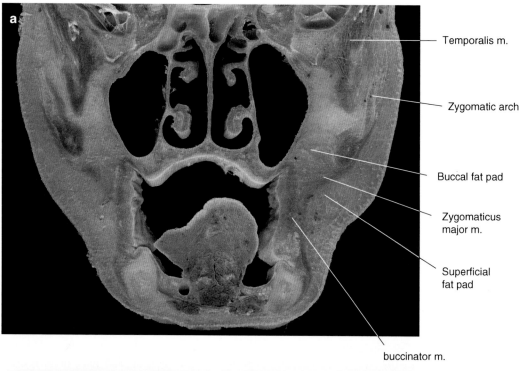

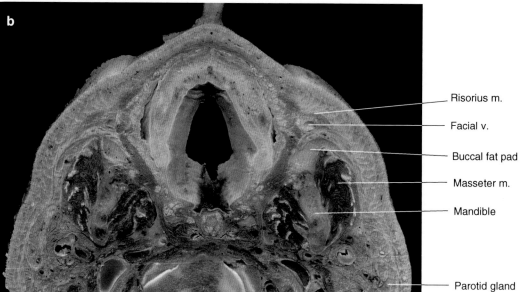

Fig. 4.27 Coronal (**a**) and transverse (**b**) sections of the head showing the buccal fat pads (Published with kind permission of © Hee-Jin Kim 2016. All rights reserved)

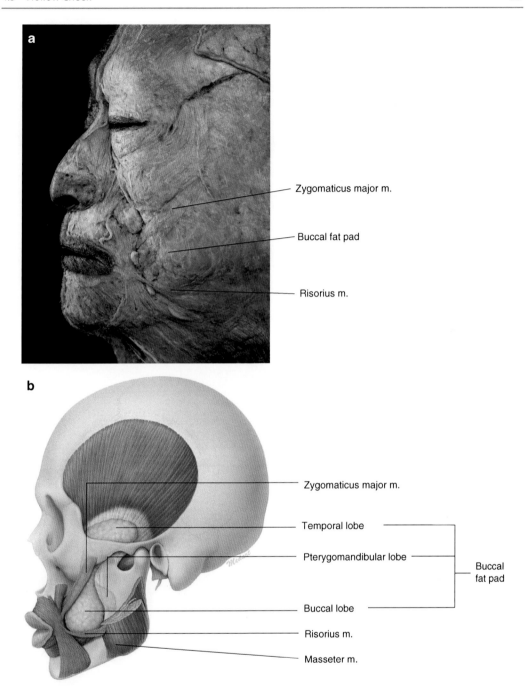

Fig. 4.28 Buccal fat pad and its lobes (**a**, **b**) (Published with kind permission of © Hee-Jin Kim 2016. All rights reserved)

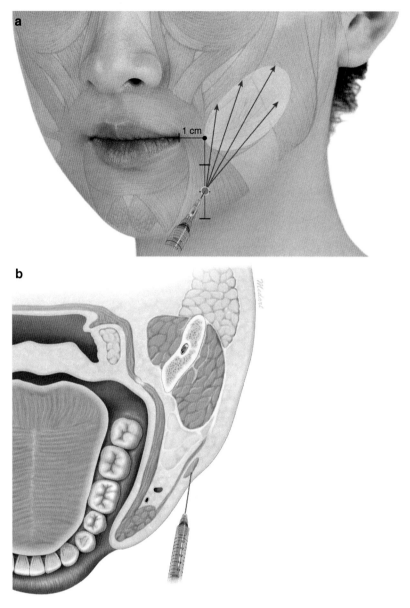

Fig. 4.29 Filler injection technique for hollow cheek (**a**) and the appropriate subcutaneous injection planes (**b**) (Published with kind permission of © Kwan-Hyun Youn 2016. All rights reserved)

4.6   Subzygoma Depression

4.6.1   Clinical Anatomy

Subzygoma depression leads to a protrusion of the zygoma. Filler treatments for subzygoma depression are recommended for those who desire to have a plump face with a less pronounced zygoma (Fig. 4.30).

The masseteric cutaneous ligament forms from the inferior border of the zygomatic arch to the anterior margin of the masseter muscle (Fig. 1.25). This ligament is one of the false retaining ligament and attaches to the skin covering the SMAS and the cheek. With age, this ligament becomes lax, and the SMAS covering the masseter m. sags. This results in sagging of the overall region also.

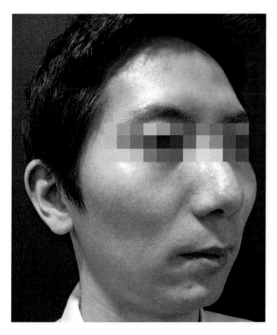

Fig. 4.30 Subzygoma depression (Published with kind permission of © Jisoo Kim 2016. All rights reserved)

4.6.2 Injection Points and Methods

Filler injection depth should be at the subcutaneous fat tissue above the masseter muscle. The area of injection can be defined by the following parameters: zygomatic arch (upper), middle 1/2 of the masseter m. (lower), and anterior and posterior border of the masseter m. (anterior and posterior, respectively). The filler injection should proceed so as to create a smooth gradation from the most sunken area below the zygomatic arch to middle of the masseter muscle.

The entry point of the cannula should be placed at the point of intersection between a vertical line drawn from the lateral canthus and an oblique line drawn from the mouth corner to the tragus.

Increasing the volume for the subzygoma depression is difficult, due to the dense connective tissue beneath the skin. In this area, there are numerous tough fascial structures, and injecting massive filler may lead to unwanted undulations and bulging during animation. A possible method is to break the attachment of dense fasciae with a sharp needle and to inject the filler afterward;

however, bruising may occur and parotid duct can be injured (Fig. 4.31).

Collagen derivative such as calcium filler may be used, but HA filler is the safest.

4.7 Nose

4.7.1 Clinical Anatomy

The nose, being located at the center of the face, plays an important aesthetic role in creating balance between the eye and the mouth (Fig. 4.32). For Asians who have a relatively lower nose bridge, filler injections rather than the rhinoplasty may be a simple and effective method for nose augmentation. Although fillers have the advantages of being less invasive than surgery, fillers lose their volume over time by naturally breaking down, and periodic injections are needed to maintain its clinical outcome. Regarding safety, side effects such as contracture of the nose that may be entailed after the surgery do not pertain in filler injection procedure; however, cosmetic effects of filler treatments are limited in that filler injections cannot make the blunt nose tip sharper or reduce big nose, remove hump, and narrow a wide nose. Nonetheless, among Asian populations with high demand for nose augmentations, filler injections are often a suitable replacement for invasive surgical procedures.

Since the criteria of aesthetic appeal vary for different populations, it is difficult to state an ideal angle for the nose that is the most appealing. However, it helps to keep in mind a range of angles for the nose that gives a person an attractive look: nasofrontal angle, 115–130°; nasofacial angle, 35–40°; and nasolabial angle, 90–110° (Fig. 4.33).

Asians tend to have thicker skin and an abundant subcutaneous tissue than Caucasians. From a cosmetic perspective, the presence of an abundant soft tissue of the nose helps to minimize the undulating appearance that is more prone to occur in Caucasians. When treating special cases such as a hooked nose, the physician should be aware that the rhinion is the thinnest area of the dorsum of the nose.

Fig. 4.31 Filler injection techniques for subzygoma depression (**a**) and the appropriate subcutaneous injection planes (**b**) (Published with kind permission of © Kwan-Hyun Youn 2016. All rights reserved)

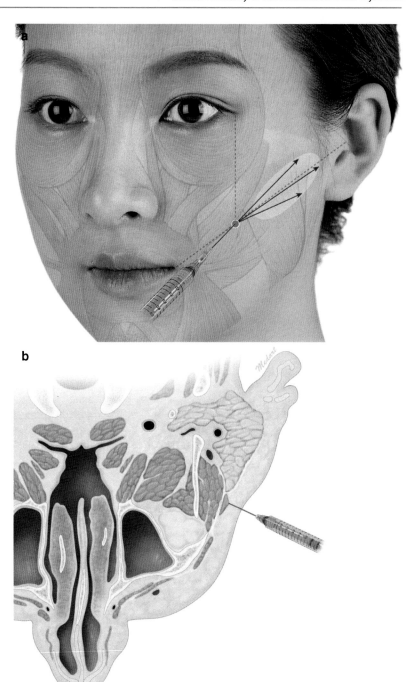

From a clinical perspective, a thick subcutaneous tissue in Asian populations is a point of greater caution because an improper injection may lead to improper intravascular injections of filler products within the subcutaneous layer.

The soft tissue of the nose consists of the skin, the superficial fatty layer, the fibromuscular layer, the deep fatty layer, and the periosteum or the perichondrium (Fig. 4.34). The fibromuscular layer is located between the superficial and deep fatty layers. Muscles near the nose are interconnected by SMAS (superficial musculoaponeurotic system) enclosing the face.

Fig. 4.32 Anthropologic landmarks on nose (Published with kind permission of © Kwan-Hyun Youn 2016. All rights reserved)

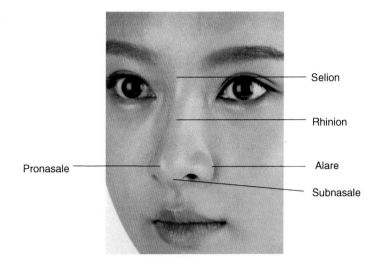

Selion

Rhinion

Pronasale

Alare

Subnasale

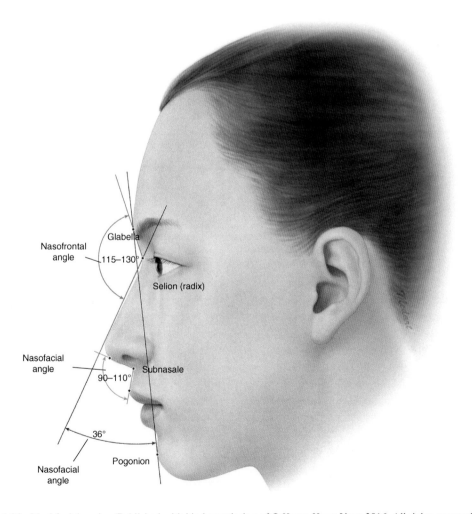

Glabella

Nasofrontal angle

115–130°

Selion (radix)

Nasofacial angle

90–110°   Subnasale

36°

Pogonion

Nasofacial angle

Fig. 4.33 Ideal facial angles (Published with kind permission of © Kwan-Hyun Youn 2016. All rights reserved)

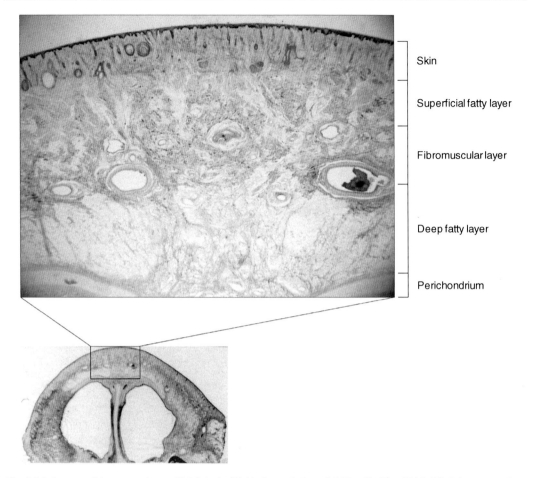

Fig. 4.34 Layers of the external nose (Published with kind permission of © Hee-Jin Kim 2016. All rights reserved)

It is known that the main arteries of the dorsum of the nose are located at the level of the superficial or deep fatty layers. However, at the lower portion of the dorsum of the nose, the dorsal nasal arterial branches are located adjacent the fibromuscular layer and the deep fatty layer (Fig. 4.34). On the other hand, at the upper portion of the dorsum of the nose (bony nose), the dorsal nasal a. run at the level of the superficial fatty layer just above the fibromuscular layer (Fig. 4.35).

Paranasal muscles include (1) the procerus m., (2) the nasalis m., (3) the depressor septi nasi muscle, and (4) dilator naris vestibularis and anterioris muscles of the nasal ala. In addition to the muscles stated previously, there are other muscles attached to the nasal ala (Fig. 4.36).

1. Procerus muscle: The procerus m. is a small muscle that arises from the nasal bone and the lateral cartilage of the nose and attaches to the skin at the radix and glabella. At this point, the muscle fibers of the procerus m. intermingle with muscle fibers of the frontalis. The procerus m. is responsible for pulling on the medial portion of the eyebrow and forming a transverse wrinkle of the glabella.

2. Nasalis muscle: The nasalis m. is formed by the transverse part and the alar part. The transverse part of the nasalis m. in a triangular shape originates from the canine fossa of the maxilla and inserts into the lateral cartilage of the nose. The alar part is a square-shaped muscle that arises from the maxilla above the maxillary lateral incisor and inserts into the lower portion of the alar cartilage. The transverse and alar parts are responsible for the narrowing of the nostrils by the contraction of the nasal aperture and widening of the nostrils, respectively.

3. Depressor septi nasi muscle: The depressor septi nasi m. is located deep within the lip. It

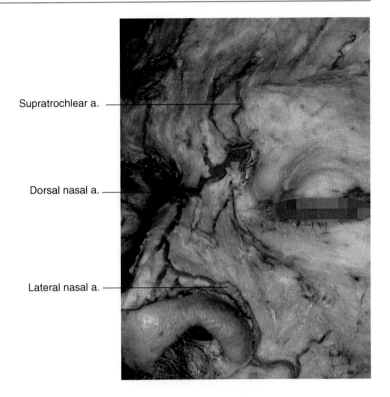

Supratrochlear a.

Dorsal nasal a.

Lateral nasal a.

originated from the incisive fossa of the maxilla and inserts into the mobile portion of nasal septum and intermingles with the deep muscle fibers of the orbicularis oris muscle. This muscle acts for pulling down the tip of the nose as to enlarge the nostrils.

4. The dilator naris vestibularis muscle is located between the external and vestibular skin of the alar lobule. Its muscle fibers radiate along the dome-shaped nasal vestibule. The dilator naris anterior muscle originates from the frontal surfaces of the lateral half of the lateral crus and the accessory alar cartilage adjacent to the lateral crus.

In addition to the muscles stated above, 90 % of the levator labii superioris alaeque nasi m. and 28 % of the zygomaticus minor m. are attached to the nasal ala (Fig. 4.37).

The filler treatment must proceed with a full awareness of the arteries and veins distributing the nose. Although rare, there are cases when intravascular injection leads to problems caused by filler products in surrounding tissues. Symptoms that follow can be divided into the intravascular embolism and the extravascular compression. The use of a cannula is advised to reduce chances of intravascular injection.

The major arteries of the nose consist of the lateral nasal a. arising from the facial a. and the dorsal nasal a. arising from the ophthalmic artery. The arteriovenous anastomosis that results from the branches of the lateral nasal a. and the dorsal nasal a. is a characteristic anatomical feature of the external nose (Figs. 4.38 and 4.39). Furthermore, the columella branches that arise from the superior labial a. distribute at the tip of the nose (Fig. 4.40). In addition to the lateral nasal a., the inferior alar a. traverses below the nasal ala. Overall, the lateral nasal and dorsal nasal arteries are largely responsible for arterial blood supply to the tip of the nose. Branches of the dorsal nasal and the angular arteries distribute at the dorsum of the nose (Figs. 4.39 and 4.40).

The dorsal nasal a. is slender and, as stated before, run at the level of the deep fatty layer at the lower dorsum of the nose. However, at the upper portion of the dorsum of the nose, the dorsal nasal a. tends to be located at the superficial fatty layer of the procerus muscle. The dorsal nasal a. originates from the ophthalmic a.; hence, it tends to run along the

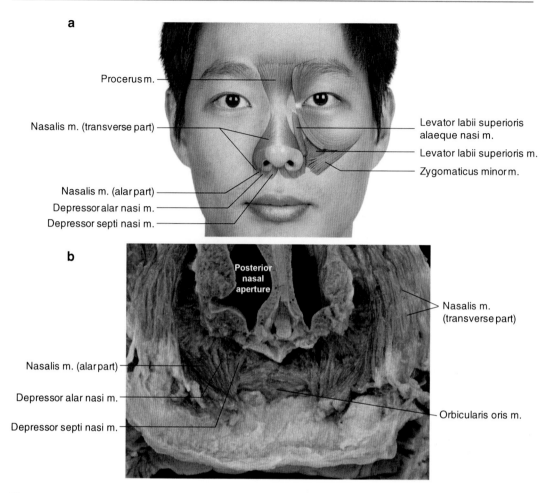

Fig. 4.36 Perinasal musculature (**a**) and a specimen revealing the detailed muscles around the nostril and nasal septum (**b**), posterior view (Published with kind permission of © Kwan-Hyun Youn 2016. All rights reserved)

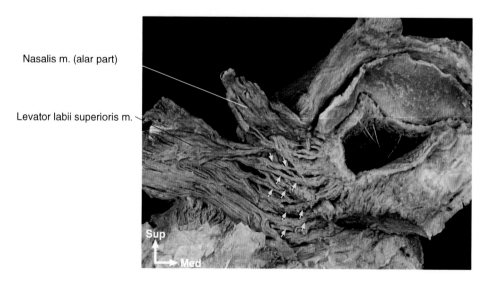

Fig. 4.37 The attachment of the levator labii superioris muscle to the nasal ala in the posterior aspect. Some deeper muscle fibers of the levator labii superioris (*arrows*) are attached to the vestibular skin of the nasal lobule (Published with kind permission of © Hee-Jin Kim 2016. All rights reserved)

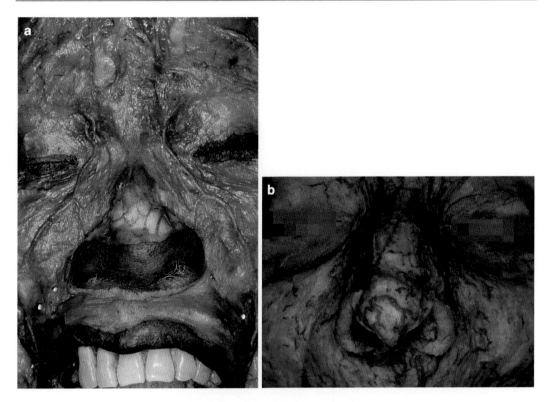

Fig. 4.38 Arterial supply on the midface and nose (**a**) and arteriovenous anastomosis of the tip of the nose (**b**) (Published with kind permission of © Hee-Jin Kim 2016. All rights reserved)

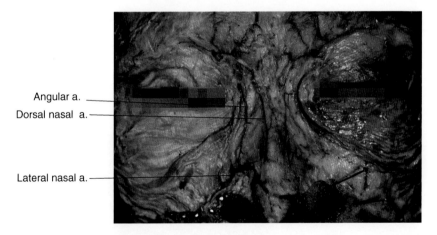

Angular a.
Dorsal nasal a.
Lateral nasal a.

Fig. 4.39 Dorsal nasal artery of the dorsum of the nose (Published with kind permission of © Hee-Jin Kim 2016. All rights reserved)

sides of the dorsum of the nose (Fig. 4.39). Small communicating branches from bilateral dorsal nasal a. are observed at the dorsum of the nose (78 % of the cases). Especially, it is memorable that the cases in which the dorsal nasal a. from one side crosses the midline of the nose and mainly supplies the opposite side can be found (21.6 % of Asian cases).

Furthermore, as shown in Fig. 4.35, a case that a relatively thick tortuous arterial branch from the

ophthalmic a. emerges from the upper medial canthal area and runs along the lateral aspect of the dorsum of the nose and then communicates with the lateral nasal a. can also be seen. In this case, injecting fillers using a needle into a point deviating lateral to the radix may be highly dangerous; therefore, aspiration should be performed prior to the injection.

The columellar branches from the superior labial a. entered the columella via the columello-

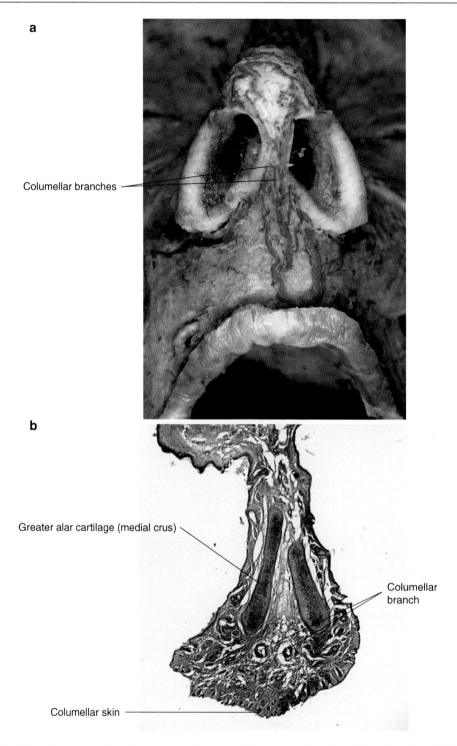

Fig. 4.40 Columellar branches from the superior labial artery (**a**) and coronal section of the columella (middle of the columella (×10)) (**b**) (Published with kind permission of © Hee-Jin Kim 2016. All rights reserved)

labial junction and distribute to the base of the nose. These branches proceeded to the medial crus of the lower lateral cartilage at the midline, at the basal and posterior portions of the septum. These vessels travel closer to the medial crus than the epidermis and locate at the level of the deep fatty layer of the infratip of the nose (Figs. 4.40 and 4.41).

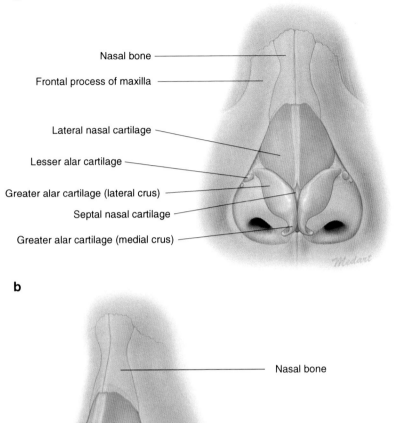

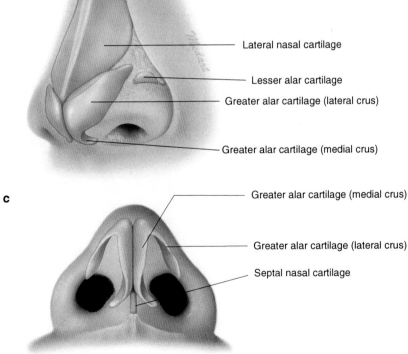

Fig. 4.41 Cartilage of the nose (**a** frontal view, **b** oblique view, **c** basal view) (Published with kind permission of © Kwan-Hyun Youn 2016. All rights reserved)

However, as these vessels run close to the tip of the nose, they give off many fine arterial branches into both the superficial and deep fatty layers of the nose. When injecting fillers for columellar augmentation, the needle entry should be done deep to the skin at the tip of the nose. Deep columellar injections toward to the medial crus are highly advised (Fig. 4.40).

4.7.2 Injection Points and Methods

4.7.2.1 Dorsum of the Nose

The injection plane of the filler with a cannula should be at the level of the supraperichondrial and supraperiosteal layer. The entry point of the cannula should be made at the infratip lobule. Beginning from the sellion (deepest point of the radix), the augmentation for dorsum of the nose should follow with the retrograde thread injection technique (Figs. 4.41, 4.42, 4.43, and 4.44).

4.7.2.2 Columella

For the columellar augmentation, the cannula should be located between the medial crus of the lateral alar cartilage and the anterior nasal spine. The insertion point of the cannula should be made at the infratip lobule.

The HA filler is the most appropriate filler for nose augmentations since it can be an easily

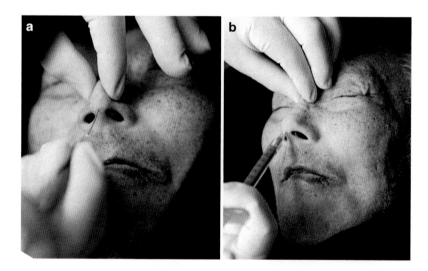

Fig. 4.42 Filler injection for nose augmentation (**a, b**) (Published with kind permission of © Hee-Jin Kim 2016. All rights reserved)

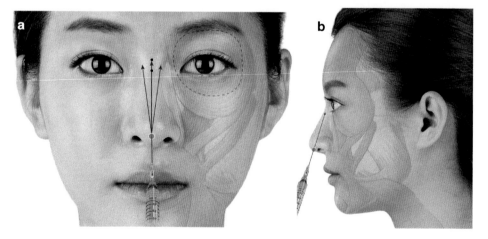

Fig. 4.43 Filler injection technique for nose augmentation (**a** frontal view, **b** lateral view) (Published with kind permission of © Kwan-Hyun Youn 2016. All rights reserved)

a

b

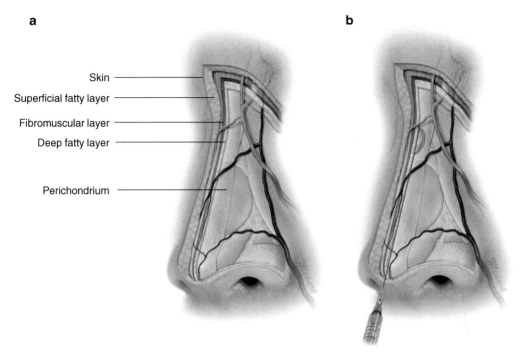

Skin

Superficial fatty layer

Fibromuscular layer

Deep fatty layer

Perichondrium

Fig. 4.44 Anatomical layers of the external nose (**a**) and appropriate plane for filler injection on dorsum of the nose (**b**)

correctable material when side effects occur. Furthermore, the use of a biphasic HA filler with a large particle size is recommended than a monophasic HA filler to minimize the risk of intravascular injection of filler mass. Fillers with a large particle size would be more suitable among various products of biphasic fillers. Although gel-type monophasic fillers tend to last longer, their properties of water absorption may lead to the side effect of a widening of the dorsum of the nose. If calcium hydroxylapatite fillers are injected, it is hardly correctable and provides little buffer room when lumps will occur in relatively thin skin area or dorsum and columella line will be not at the proper line. So HA fillers are strongly recommended.

The Anatomy of the Intercanthal Vein in Asians

Many venous branches embedded at the subcutaneous layer of the radix and glabella. Among the complicated venous networks, intercanthal v. (ICV) located at the subcutaneous layer can be observed in every case (Fig. 4.45). The intercanthal v. is found to be located above and below the level of the intercanthal line that connects the medial canthi on both sides (70.7 % of the cases).

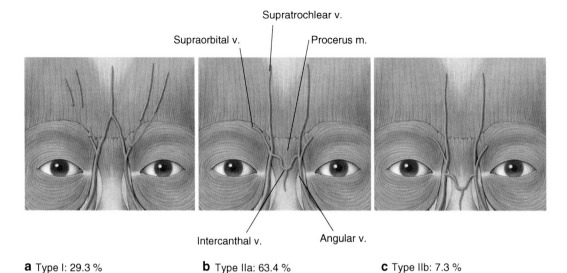

a Type I: 29.3 %   **b** Type IIa: 63.4 %   **c** Type IIb: 7.3 %

Fig. 4.45 Distribution patterns and classification of the intercanthal vein (ICV). (**a**) Type I, near the midsagittal line, a single STV divides into two branches and each of the branches of the STV runs obliquely downward close to the medial canthus to meet the SOV, ultimately becoming the AV. (**b**) Type IIa, the ICV is located above the intercanthal line (ICL). (**c**) Type IIb, the ICV is located below the ICL in the nasoglabellar area (Published with kind permission of © Kwan-Hyun Youn 2016. All rights reserved)

Suggested Reading

Physical Anthropological Traits in Asians

1. Chung MS, Kim HJ, Kang HS, Chung IH. Locational relationship of the supraorbital notch or foramen and infraorbital and mental foramina in Koreans. Acta Anat. 1995;154:162–6.
2. Kim SH, Whang E, Choi HG, Shin DH, Uhm KI, Chung H, Song WC, Koh KS. Analysis of the midface, focusing on the nose: an anthropometric study in young Koreans. J Craniofac Surg. 2010;21:1941–4.
3. Koh KS, Shon HJ, Rhee EK, Park SJ, Kim HJ, Han SH, Chung RH. Anthropological study on the facial flatness of Korean from the historic to the modern period. Korean J Phys Anthrop. 1999;12:211–21.
4. Rho NK, Chang YY, Chao YY, Furuyama N, Huang P, Kerscher M, Kim HJ, Park JY, Peng P, Rummaneethorn P, Rzany B, Sundaram H, Wong CH, Yang Y, Prasetyo AD. Consensus recommendations for optimal augmentation of the Asian face with hyaluronic acid and calcium hydroxylapatite fillers. Plast Reconstr Surg. 2015;136(5):940–56.
5. Song WC, Kim SH, Paik DJ, Han SH, Hu KS, Kim HJ, Koh KS. Location of the infra-orbital and mental foramen with reference to the soft tissue landmarks. Plast Reconstr Surg. 2007;120:1343–7.
6. Youn KH, Kim YC, Hu KS, Song WC, Kim HJ, Koh KS. An art anatomical study of the facial profile of Korean. Korean J Phys Anthrop. 2002;15:251–62.

Muscles of the Face and Neck

7. Choi DY, Kim JS, Youn KH, Hur MS, Kim JS, Hu KS, Kim HJ. Clinical anatomic considerations of the zygomaticus minor muscle based on the morphology and insertion pattern. Dermatol Surg. 2014;40(8):858–63.
8. Hu KS, Jin GC, Youn KH, Kwak HH, Koh KS, Fontaine C, Kim HJ. An anatomic study of the bifid zygomaticus major muscle. J Craniofac Surg. 2008;19(2):534–5.
9. Hur MS, Hu KS, Park JT, Youn KH, Kim HJ. New anatomical insight of the levator labii superioris alaeque nasi and the transverse part of the nasalis. Surg Radiol Anat. 2010;32(8):753–6.
10. Hur MS, Hu KS, Youn KH, Song WC, Abe S, Kim HJ. New anatomical profile of the nasal musculature: dilator naris vestibularis, dilator naris anterior, and alar part of the nasalis. Clin Anat. 2011;24(2):162–7.
11. Hur MS, Youn KH, Hu KS, Song WC, Koh KS, Fontaine C, Kim HJ. New anatomic considerations on the levator labii superioris related with the nasal ala. J Craniofac Surg. 2010;21(1):258–60.
12. Hwang WS, Hur MS, Hu KS, Song WC, Koh KS, Baik HS, Kim ST, Kim HJ, Lee KJ. Surface anatomy of the lip elevator muscles for the treatment of gummy smile using botulinum toxin. Angle Orthod. 2009;79(1):70–7.
13. Park JT, Youn KH, Hu KS, Kim HJ. Medial muscular band of the orbicularis oculi muscle. J Craniofac Surg. 2012;23(1):195–7.
14. Park JT, Youn KH, Hur MS, Hu KS, Kim HJ, Kim HJ. Malaris muscle, the lateral muscular band

of orbicularis oculi muscle. J Craniofac Surg. 2011;22(2):659–62.

15. Shim KS, Hu KS, Kwak HH, Youn KH, Koh KS, Fontaine C, Kim HJ. An anatomy of the insertion of the zygomaticus major muscle in human focused on the muscle arrangement at the mouth corner. Plast Reconstr Surg. 2008;121(2):466–73.

16. Youn KH, Park JT, Park DS, Koh KS, Kim HJ, Paik DJ. Morphology of the zygomaticus minor and its relationship with the orbicularis oculi muscle. J Craniofac Surg. 2012;23(2):546–8.

Vessels of the Face and Neck

17. Jung DH, Kim HJ, Koh KS, Oh CS, Kim KS, Yoon JH, Chung IH. Arterial supply of the nasal tip in Asians. Laryngoscope. 2000;110(2):308–11.

18. Kim YS, Choi DY, Gil YC, Hu KS, Tansatit T, Kim HJ. The anatomical origin and course of the angular artery regarding its clinical implications. Dermatol Surg. 2014;40(10):1070–6.

19. Koh KS, KIM HJ, Oh CS, Chung IH. Branching patterns and symmetry of the course of the facial artery in Koreans. Int J Oral Max Surg. 2003;32(4):414–8.

20. Kwak HH, Hu KS, Youn KH, Jin KH, Shim KS, Fontaine C, Kim HJ. Topographic relationship between the muscle bands of the zygomaticus major muscle and the facial artery. Surg Radiol Anat. 2006;28(5):477–80.

21. Kwak HH, Jo JB, Hu KS, Oh CS, Koh KS, Chung IH, Kim HJ. Topography of the third portion of the maxillary artery via the transantral approach in Asians. J Craniofac Surg. 2010;21(4):1284–9.

22. Lee HJ, Kang IW, Won SY, Lee JG, Hu KS, Tansatit T, Kim HJ. Description of a novel anatomical venous structure in the nasoglabellar area. J Craniofac Surg. 2014;25(2):633–5.

23. Lee JG, Yang HM, Choi YJ, Favero V, Kim YS, Hu KS, Kim HJ. Facial arterial depth and layered relationship with facial musculatures. Plast Reconstr Surg. 2015;135:437–44.

24. Lee SH, Gil YC, Choi YJ, Tansatit T, Kim HJ, Hu KS. Topographic anatomy of superior labial artery for dermal filler injection. Plast Reconstr Surg. 2015;135:445–50.

25. Lee SH, Lee M, Kim HJ. Anatomy-based image-processing analysis for the running pattern of the perioral artery for minimally invasive surgery. Br J Oral Max Surg. 2014;52(8):688–92.

26. Lee YI, Yang HM, Pyeon HJ, Lee HK, Kim HJ. Anatomical and histological study of the arterial distribution in the columellar area, and the clinical implications. Surg Radiol Anat. 2014;36(7):669–74.

27. Park KH, Kim YK, Woo SJ, Kang SW, Lee WK, Choi KS, Kwak HW, Yoon IH, Huh K, Kim JW. Iatrogenic occlusion of the ophthalmic artery after cosmetic facial filler injections: a national survey by the Korean Retina Society. JAMA Ophthalmol. 2014;132(6):714–23.

28. Yang HM, Lee JG, Hu KS, Gil YC, Choi YJ, Lee HK, Kim HJ. New anatomical insights of the course and branching patterns of the facial artery: clinical implications regarding injectable treatments to the nasolabial fold and nasojugal groove. Plast Reconstr Surg. 2014;133(5):1077–82.

29. Yang HM, Lee YI, Lee JG, Choi YJ, Lee HJ, Lee SH, Hu KS, Kim HJ. Topography of superficial arteries on the face. J Phys Anthropol. 2013;26:131–40.

Peripheral Nerves of the Face and Neck

30. Hu KS, Kwak HH, Song WC, Kang HJ, Kim HC, Fontaine C, Kim HJ. Branching patterns of the infraorbital nerve and topography within the infraorbital space. J Craniofac Surg. 2006;17(6):1111–5.

31. Hu KS, Kwak J, Koh KS, Abe S, Fontaine C, Kim HJ. Topographic distribution area of the infraorbital nerve. Surg Radiol Anat. 2007;29(5):383–8.

32. Yang HM, Won SY, Kim HJ, Hu KS. Sihler staining study of anastomosis between the facial and trigeminal nerves in the ocular area and its clinical implications. Muscle Nerve. 2013;48(4):545–50.

33. Yang HM, Won SY, Kim HJ, Hu KS. Sihler's staining study of the infraorbital nerve and its clinical complication. J Craniofac Surg. 2014;25(6):2209–13.

Clinical Anatomy of the Lower Face for Filler Injection

5

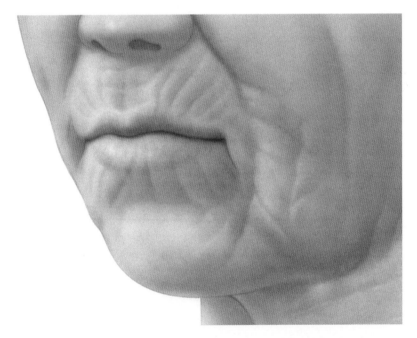

Jisoo Kim, MD, MS, Hong-Ki Lee, MD, PhD, and Hee-Jin Kim, DDS, PhD (Illustrated by Kwan-Hyun Youn)

© Springer Science+Business Media Singapore 2016
H.-J. Kim et al., *Clinical Anatomy of the Face for Filler and Botulinum Toxin Injection*,
DOI 10.1007/978-981-10-0240-3_5

5.1 Lip

Filler injection on the lips is often conducted to reduce, to refine the contour, and to have voluptuous lip. More specifically, filler treatment can reduce the presence of vertical lip wrinkles (smoker lines) that start on the vermilion border as an aging.

5.1.1 Clinical Anatomy

The vermilion border is the red border marking the periphery of the lip. The cupid bow is the heart-shaped dimple centrally located above the upper lip. The vertical groove between the nose and the mouth is called the philtrum. The oral commissure (cheilion) is located at the corner of the mouth where the upper lip and the lower lip meet (Fig. 5.1). With age, the vermilion border becomes dimmer, while the smoker lines become more pronounced. Overall, aging leads to a reduction of lip volume resulting in the appearance of a thinner, flaccid lip.

A frontal view of the lip shows that the lip is composed of an intermediate zone—red portion—that lies between the cutaneous portion and the mucous portion. The vermilion border can also be defined as the region between the cutaneous portion and the intermediate zone. The mucous portion can be further divided into the dry mucosa and the wet mucosa with the junction between the two being defined as the dry-wet mucosal junction. Located directly below the

mucous portion are the superior labial a., the inferior labial a., the mental n., and the labial gland. They are located on the deeper layer than the orbicularis oris m. (Figs. 5.2 and 5.3).

5.1.2 Injection Points and Methods

The lip is highly sensitive to pain; therefore, the use of nerve block anesthesia is recommended when a topical anesthetic ointment does not suffice. The infraorbital n. and the mental n. innervate the upper and lower lip, respectively. A definitive knowledge of the nerve pathways and branching points must accompany the anesthetic procedure (Fig. 5.3).

The use of a hard filler on the lips leads to visible irregularity of the lips and irritation to the patient; therefore, the use of soft fillers is advised. If the goal of filler injections is to accentuate the contour of the lip, the treatment should proceed with injecting the filler along the vermilion border into the dermal and subdermal layer. When trying to increase volume, the filler should be injected into the submucosal or intramuscular layer below the mucous portion of the lip (Fig. 5.4). Injecting the filler into the dry-wet mucosa junction can help to reverse the inversion of the lips caused by aging. It is best to avoid injecting deeply into the muscle layer from the wet mucosa, because of the potential risk of damaging the superior and inferior labial a. with understanding the anatomical location of the arteries of the lip.

It is possible to use a needle or cannula. When trying to increase the overall volume of the lips, the

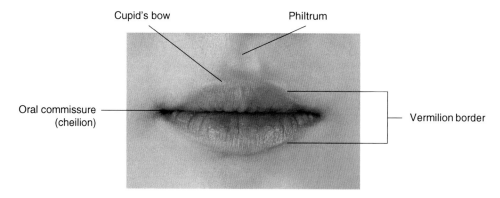

Fig. 5.1 Lip (Published with kind permission of © Kwan-Hyun Youn 2016. All rights reserved)

Fig. 5.2 Sagittal section of the lip (Published with kind permission of © Hee-Jin Kim 2016. All rights reserved)

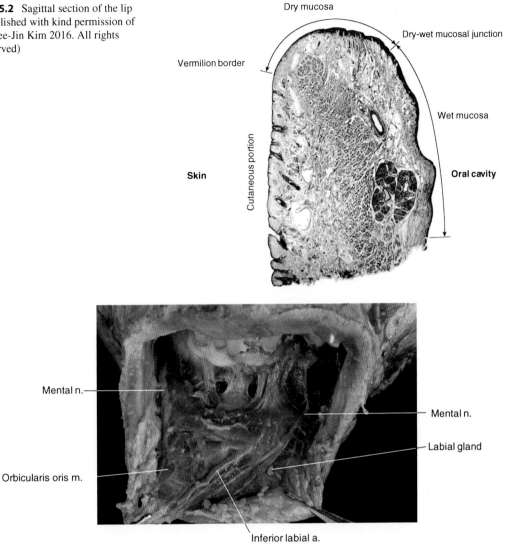

Fig. 5.3 A dissection of the lower lip (Published with kind permission of © Hee-Jin Kim 2016. All rights reserved)

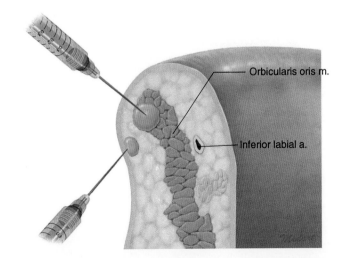

Fig. 5.4 Filler injection technique for lip volume and lip contour (Published with kind permission of © Kwan-Hyun Youn 2016. All rights reserved)

Fig. 5.5 Filler injection techniques for lip augmentation (**a** needle injection for lip line, **b** needle injection for lip volume, **c** injection point for the cannula, published with kind permission of © Kwan-Hyun Youn 2016. All rights reserved)

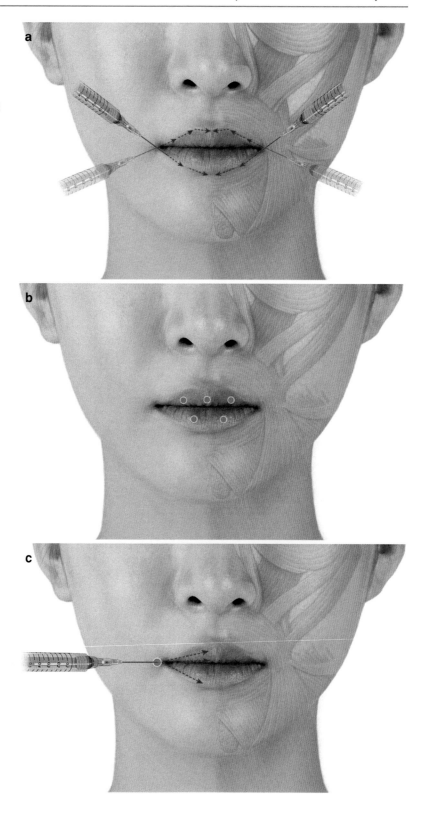

use of a cannula is advised. The area around oral commissure can be an insertion point for the cannula. The use of a needle is advised when injecting fillers into specific points at the mucous portion of the lip with cutaneous approach to prevent bleeding from highly vascular mucosa (Figs. 5.5 and 5.6).

If the vertical lip lines around vermilion border are not too deep enough, injecting a HA filler into the vermilion border may suffice in reducing the wrinkles by accentuating the vermilion border. However, if the vertical lip lines are deep, it may be necessary to have a filler injection into the dermis of each wrinkle. In this case, injection should be cautious not to make uneven surface due to superficial injection. Combination usage

of botulinum toxin with dermal injection of filler can increase the effectiveness of filler treatment.

5.1.3 Side Effects

The superior labial a. and v. and inferior labial a. and v. traverse the lip. The lateral corner of the mouth is the reference point by which the facial a. is divided into the superior labial a. and the inferior labial a. The superior labial a. follows the upper lip, and the inferior labial a. branches about 1.5 cm inferior to the lower lip, deeply passes the middle ½ area of the DAO, and runs along with the mental crease to give off the branches into the lower lip (Fig. 5.7).

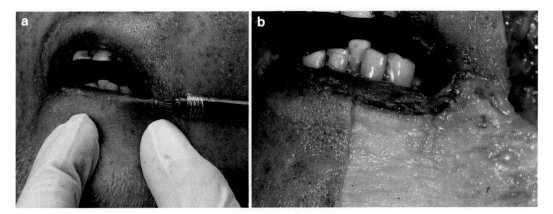

Fig. 5.6 Filler injection on the cadaveric lip (**a**) and the properly located filler product along the vermilion border (**b**) on subdermal layer (Published with kind permission of © Hee-Jin Kim 2016. All rights reserved)

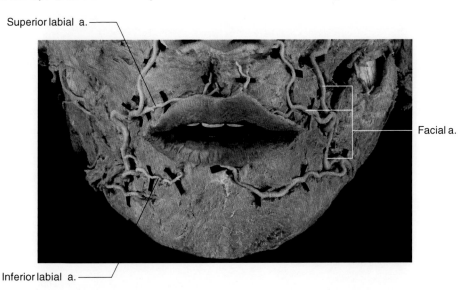

Fig. 5.7 Superior and inferior labial artery of the lip (Published with kind permission of © Hee-Jin Kim 2016. All rights reserved)

Topographic Anatomy of the Labial Artery
The superior labial a. arises from the facial a. near the oral commissure and follows the vermilion border of the upper lip. When it reaches the philtrum, it separates into the columellar branch. The topographical anatomy of the inferior labial a. is more complicated as it does not follow a specifically designated path; however, it commonly follows the vermilion border of the lower lip or runs past the center of the chin.

1. Relative location of the labial arteries

The facial a. can be classified according to its branching point and its end point; however, it commonly twists around the antegonial notch of the masseter m. and flows up the mandible. The facial a. further separates into the inferior labial a. and the superior labial a. and flows toward the nasal ala. The perioral (PO) line, drawn from the AGN to the nasal ala, serves as a reference marker for the relative locations of arteries that traverse the oral cavity.

The perioral a. can be classified into an oblique and vertical pattern. A perioral a. that follows a vertical pattern does not follow the PO line. The alar branch arises from the superior labial a. and flows in a vertical pattern (Fig. 5.8).

2. Superior labial artery

The superior labial a. arises from the facial a. in a ramification area in the shape of a square with 15 mm sides. As it approaches the vermilion border, the superior labial a. traverses through the orbicularis m. or between the orbicularis oris m. and the labial mucosa (Fig. 5.9). The superior labial a., before reaching the cupid bow, flows below the vermilion border. The columellar branches arise from the superior labial a. near the philtrum or merge with the superior labial a. coming from the opposite side. The columellar branches traverse parallel to the central line of the face and branch out into superficial and deep branches that traverse above and below the orbicularis oris. Usually, if the superficial branch arises from the superior labial a., the deep branch arises from the superior labial a. coming from the opposite side. There are cases when both of the superficial and deep branches arise from a single superior labial a. with the artery com-

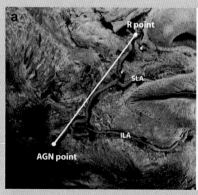
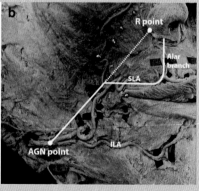
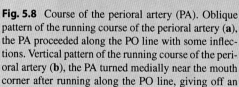

Fig. 5.8 Course of the perioral artery (PA). Oblique pattern of the running course of the perioral artery (**a**), the PA proceeded along the PO line with some inflections. Vertical pattern of the running course of the perioral artery (**b**), the PA turned medially near the mouth corner after running along the PO line, giving off an alar branch parallel to the facial sagittal midline. PO line: the perioral line connecting the antegonial notch (AGN point) and the ramification point of the lateral nasal artery and the inferior alar branch (R point, published with kind permission of © Hee-Jin Kim 2016. All rights reserved)

Fig. 5.9 Ramification of the superior labial artery (Published with kind permission of © Kwan-Hyun Youn 2016. All rights reserved)

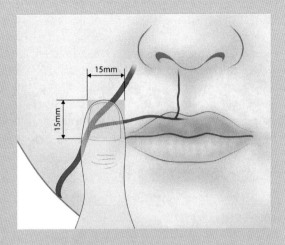

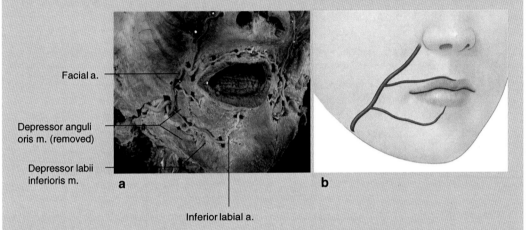

Facial a.

Depressor anguli oris m. (removed)

Depressor labii inferioris m.

a

b

Inferior labial a.

Fig. 5.10 Ramification of the inferior labial artery (Published with kind permission of © Hee-Jin Kim and Kwan-Hyun Youn 2016. All rights reserved)

ing from the opposite side and terminating without extending columellar branches.

3. Inferior labial artery

The inferior labial a. arises from the facial a. and supplies blood to the mucous membrane and to the labial gland of the lower lip. About 1–3 branches of the facial a. are observed to be the inferior labial a., and their paths are highly diverse. There is a low frequency of the inferior labial a. running parallel to the vermilion border of the lower lip; rather, it flows past the center of the chin and runs between the depressor anguli oris m. and the depressor labii inferioris m. and terminates at the mucous membrane of the lower lip (Fig. 5.10).

When injecting into the vermilion border to accentuate the contour of the upper lip, the physician must proceed with caution to avoid injecting too deeply into the muscle layer. If injected too deep, the filler may be injected into the superior labial a. When injecting into the lip for the purpose of volume augmentation, it is advised to approach from dry mucosa, not wet mucosa, because it is more likely to injure superior and inferior labial a. which are closely located in soft tissue of wet mucosa (Figs. 5.2 and 5.7).

5.2   Chin

Filler injection is a possible treatment for the patient with a retruded chin, a square chin, a short chin, or a double chin (Fig. 5.11). Filler injection may be an efficient way to create pointed chin what is colloquially known as the "V-line." Chin augmentation should be taken into consideration both of the projection and of elongation of the chin. Due to the overdeveloped mentalis m. in many Asians, the lower chin is a common target for filler and botulinum injection.

5.2.1   Clinical Anatomy

Since a retruded chin is prevalent in Asians, the demand for filler injection is relatively high. Bimaxillary protrusion, common in Asians,

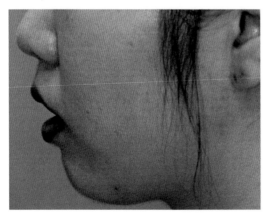

Fig. 5.11 Retruded chin (Published with kind permission of © Hong-Ki Lee 2016. All rights reserved)

causes are greater tension in closing the mouth; therefore, the hypertrophy of the mentalis m. often leads to a cobblestone appearance of the skin on the chin. Treatment of the cobblestone appearance often requires the combined usage of botulinum toxins and fillers.

The tissue layers that compose the chin can be defined as the skin, the subcutaneous tissue, the mentalis m., and the mandible. Since the layers that compose the chin are not strictly aligned, a three-dimensional approach to its anatomical composition is highly advised. Due to the medial fibers of the mentalis forming a dome-shaped chin prominence in the posterior aspect (Fig. 5.12), there is vacant space interspersed with fat and ligamentous structure between the muscle fibers (Figs. 5.3 and 5.13).

5.2.2   Injection Points and Methods

Injection layers can be above the periosteum, intramuscular, and the subcutaneous tissue. Injecting just above the periosteum minimizes the risk of an intravascular injection. When injecting into this layer, the use of hard fillers is recommended, and copious amounts of filler can be sometimes needed to create the chin shape. When space for filler injection is insufficient due to high tension of tissue, the injection can be divided into 2–3 sessions waiting for tissue expansion effect of previous filler injection. If the chin is severely retruded and the mentalis muscle is highly developed, filler injection alone is often insufficient to bring about a definite improvement of the shape due to strong contraction of the hypertrophied mentalis muscle. Hyperactive contraction of the mentalis muscle induces migration of filler material into superior direction, and duration of filler is prone to be short. As a result, the combined usage of botulinum toxin with the filler is strongly advised; in severe cases, surgical correction could be often recommended.

Prior to injecting into the chin, the degree of retrusion and the fat volume of the subcutaneous layer should be confirmed. Copious amounts of superficial fat tissue at the center of the chin on patients with mild retruded chin allow for an

Mentalis m.   Incisive labii inferioris m.

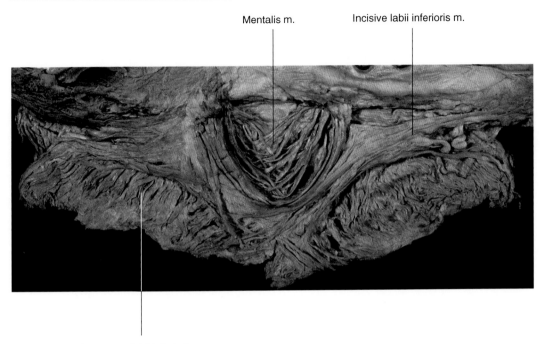

Depressor labii inferioris m.

Fig. 5.12 Medial fibers of the mentalis forming a dome-shaped chin prominence in the posterior aspect. The medial fibers of the mentalis descend anteromedially to cross together, thus forming a dome-shaped chin prominence (Published with kind permission of © Hee-Jin Kim 2016. All rights reserved)

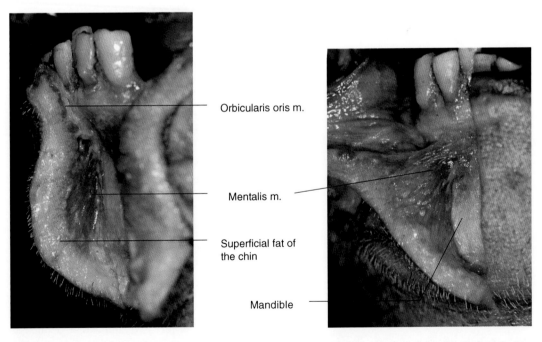

Orbicularis oris m.

Mentalis m.

Superficial fat of the chin

Mandible

Fig. 5.13 Origin and cutaneous insertion of the mentalis muscle (**a** midsagittal section of the chin, **b** frontal view, published with kind permission of © Hee-Jin Kim 2016. All rights reserved)

effective increase in chin volume via only small amount of filler injection. However, in the case of a severely recessed chin, the superficial fat tissue may be absent. In this case, filler injection into the subcutaneous fatty layer may not be the only cause of rugged surface but also cause of leaking the filler from the entry point. So injection deep onto the periosteum at the center of the chin is advised with the large volume of hard filler (Fig. 5.14). Furthermore, a caution should be paid in order to prevent a rugged surface when injecting the lateral side of the chin due to the thin subcutaneous fatty layer.

A needle is often used when injecting fillers into the chin. When the initial filler injection into the space between the chin and the mentalis m. is insufficient to create enough projection, additional injection into the subcutaneous layer could be performed. When targeting a larger area of the chin, the use of a cannula may be effective to reduce bruising. The injection layers of the cannula can be similar with the needle injection: over the periosteum, intramuscular, and subcutaneous. Injection could perform either from the center of the chin to the lateral margin or from the lateral margin to the center of the chin (Fig. 5.15). Jaw line rejuvenation may have to accompany the chin augmentation. Filler injec-

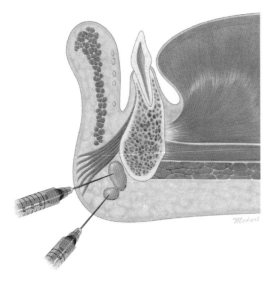

Fig. 5.14 Filler injection plane for chin augmentation (Published with kind permission of © Kwan-Hyun Youn 2016. All rights reserved)

tion into the chin may cause a dented appearance in the prejowl area—the border between the chin and the mandibular body. In order to refine the jaw line, fillers should be injected into the tip of the chin and be extended toward the mandibular angle (Fig. 5.16).

When injecting below the tip of the chin, the filler may leak into the surface of the platysma muscle. This is the case that the injected filler product leaks through the vulnerable space within the mentalis m. or along the subcutaneous fatty layer. In this case, instead of the lower margin, the needle should place in the direction of the anterior aspect of the mandible. Furthermore, it is best for physician to confirm the amount of filler injected with his/her free fingers.

Prior to the chin filler augmentation, physician should take into consideration the general contour on the patient's face, facial symmetry, jaw line symmetry, mentolabial creases, and jowl (Fig. 5.17). If these points are not evaluated before the procedure, the physician battings the risk of aggravating the patient's facial asymmetry.

5.2.3 Side Effects

Although the chin harbors the mental a. that passes through the mental foramen and the inferior labial a. from the facial a., the chin is a relatively safe area for filler injection. However, since the usage of a needle can lead to severe bruising, the procedure should not be taken lightly. In rare cases, the inferior labial a. originates from the submental a. at the submental triangle and supplies the lower lip. In this case, severe bruising or arterial injury may occur after filler injection.

Tip: Chin Filler Augmentation
The high demand for the chin filler augmentation in Asian populations could attribute to the prevalence of a recessed chin in Asians and the increasing demand for a "V-line" face.

A retruded or recessed chin can be defined as a lack of projection of the tip on the chin. Not only a retruded chin accentuates the protrusion of the mouth but also produces an angry or unsatis-

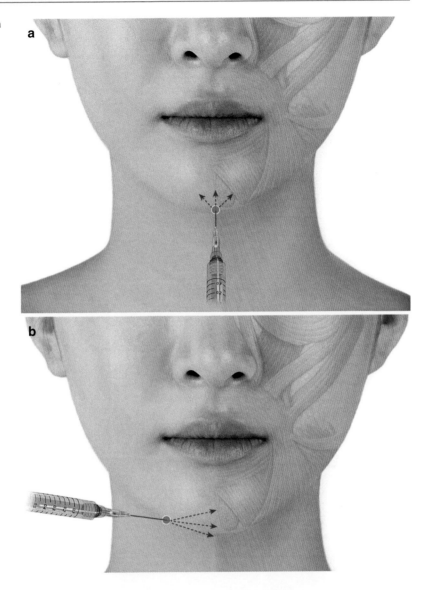

Fig. 5.15 Filler injection techniques for the chin augmentation using needle (**a**) and cannula (**b**) (Published with kind permission of © Kwan-Hyun Youn 2016. All rights reserved)

fied appearance. For certain patients, the degree of retrusion may also influence the patient's jaw mobility. Although, in the past, maxillofacial surgery was the main method of treatment, the development of filler injection techniques has allowed many invasive surgical procedures to be replaced by non-invasive filler treatments.

Prior to the filler injection, a clinical evaluation of the patient's oral and maxillofacial condition is an important step to decide whether the patient's demands can be met by filler augmentation or the orthodontic treatment should be required. A quick method for evaluating the degree of retru-

sion is to observe the Ricketts aesthetic line from the nose tip (pronasale) to the most anterior point of the chin (pogonion) (Fig. 5.18). An ideal case in Asian is when the Ricketts line completely aligns with a line drawn from the nose to the vermilion border of the lower lip. The extent of the treatment should be evaluated based on the shortage of chin relation to the proportion of the upper face, midface, lower face, and the length and proportion of the mandible against the lower facial dimension (Fig. 1.53). For Koreans, the lower face tends to be shorter with a ratio of 1:1:0.8 instead of 1:1:1 of the ideal western artis-

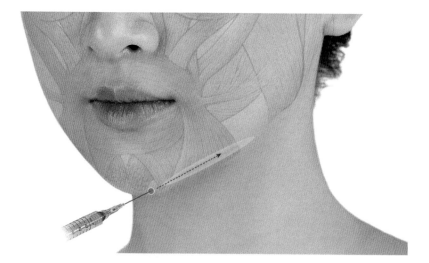

Fig. 5.16 Filler injection technique for jaw line formation after chin augmentation using cannula (Published with kind permission of © Kwan-Hyun Youn 2016. All rights reserved)

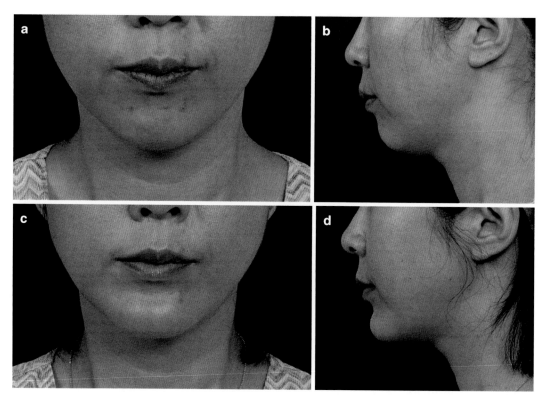

Fig. 5.17 Chin augmentation using filler before (**a**, **b**) and after (**c**, **d**) the injection (Published with kind permission of © Hong-Ki Lee 2016. All rights reserved)

tic facial ratio. Rather than adjusting the facial ratio to 1:1:1, the facial ratio should be adjusted after examining the general contour of the face.

A frontal view accompanied by a lateral view of the chin gives better insight into the projection and elongation of the patient's chin. A retruded chin does not always mean that the chin is short. In cases of long mandible with retruded chin, filler injection for the chin augmentation makes the mandible longer though yet retruded chin is corrected.

Fig. 5.18 Ricketts aesthetic line (Published with kind permission of © Kwan-Hyun Youn 2016. All rights reserved)

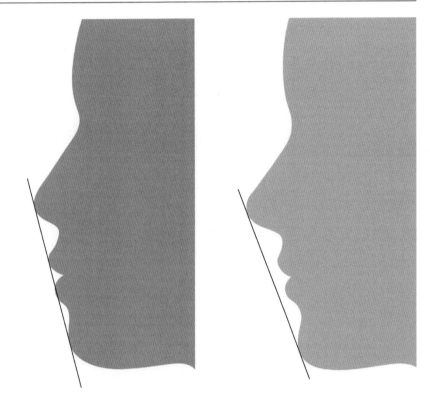

A hard filler of high viscoelasticity should be used for chin augmentation. A hardest filler of sufficient volume (2–4 cc) among calcium hydroxylapatite or HA filler should be used. All fillers that have been released until recently are not as hard as implants of prostheses; therefore, the filler may lose its rigidness or migrate by the action of mentalis m. over time. The position of the chin at the center of the face makes it highly susceptible to asymmetry in the case of imperfect filler injection; therefore, the centerline of the face should be marked prior to the procedure. Furthermore, after injection, the filler should be massaged to create a symmetrical look. When space at the chin is insufficient, injecting small amounts of fillers over 2–3 procedures is recommended rather than injecting a large amount of filler in a single procedure.

5.3   Perioral Wrinkles

Perioral wrinkles become more pronounced with age. Filler injection helps to reduce the visibility of perioral wrinkles.

5.3.1   Clinical Anatomy

The formation of perioral wrinkles is not only due to the direct muscle activity; rather, perioral wrinkles form due to a thinning of the skin and the decrease of the supporting tissue by the loss of fat tissue. The repeated animation of muscles and skin foldings is aggravating factors that contribute to the transition of perioral wrinkles into static wrinkles (Fig. 5.19).

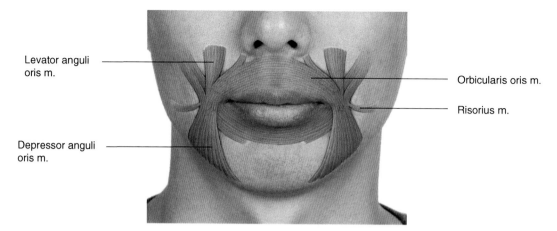

Fig. 5.19 Muscular arrangement of the perioral muscles (Published with kind permission of © Kwan-Hyun Youn 2016. All rights reserved)

5.3.2 Injection Points and Methods

When treating perioral wrinkles, direct injection into the wrinkles is possible; however, complete rejuvenation is difficult and injection by means of the hydrolifting method is advised. The filler product should be injected into the subdermis on multiple points at a 1 cm distance from each other. A cannula or needle can be used (Figs. 5.20 and 5.21). The repeated treatment sessions are necessary, because perioral area is very dynamic.

5.3.3 Side Effects

Facial aa. and vv. traverse the perioral area, and injection below the subdermis can lead to bruise and vascular damage. Caution is required since blood vessels traverse the subdermis in areas around the winding portion of the facial a. in the lateral border of the orbicularis oris m. and in a 1.5 cm circumference around the point of division between the superior labial a. and the facial a. Soft filler should be injected lightly into the dermis (Fig. 5.21). Injection into the subdermis may lead to damaged capillaries, but the chance of damaging the facial a. is very low. Therefore, the

injection must be proceeding with caution, to not inject too deeply to prevent facial vascular damage. Sufficiently soft filler must be injected into the subdermis to avoid the formation of lumps.

5.4 Marionette Line and Jowl

Marionette lines are wrinkles descending from the labial commissure toward the chin. Marionette line makes "sad appearance," and presence of the jowl breaks smooth jaw line and aggravates prejowl sulcus, which gives the appearance of aging (Fig. 5.22).

5.4.1 Clinical Anatomy

As aging occurs, jowl forms because the superficial buccal fat and the buccal fat pad droop due to gravity while the mandibular ligament stays in place. The jowl proceeds from the labial commissure and gradually becomes more pronounced in the lower chin portion. The overall effect is a bulgy chin line. The furrow that forms in front of the jowl is called the prejowl sulcus.

With aging, the buccal fat pad droops behind the risorius and depressor anguli oris muscle. As

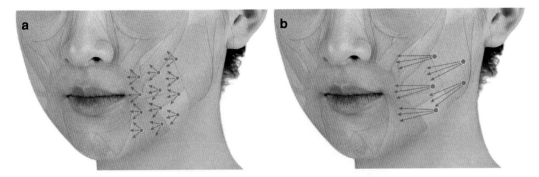

Fig. 5.20 Filler injection techniques for the perioral wrinkles using hydrolifting needle (**a**) and cannula (**b**) (Published with kind permission of © Kwan-Hyun Youn 2016. All rights reserved)

Fig. 5.21 Cadaveric filler injection for the hydrolifting using a needle and the filler product (*blue*) properly located in subdermis (Published with kind permission of © Jisoo Kim 2016. All rights reserved)

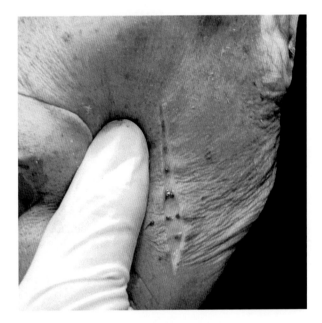

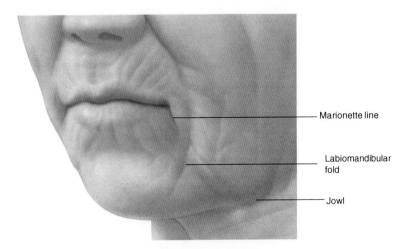

— Marionette line

— Labiomandibular fold

— Jowl

Fig. 5.22 Marionette line and jowl (Published with kind permission of © Kwan-Hyun Youn 2016. All rights reserved)

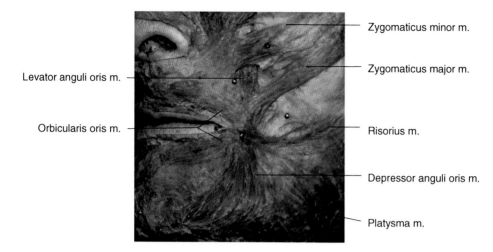

Levator anguli oris m.

Orbicularis oris m.

Zygomaticus minor m.

Zygomaticus major m.

Risorius m.

Depressor anguli oris m.

Platysma m.

Fig. 5.23 The superficial layer of the perioral muscles (Published with kind permission of © Hee-Jin KIm 2016. All rights reserved)

aging occurs and the skin and soft tissue become thinner, the lateral or posterior borders of the depressor anguli oris m. become more pronounced, while the labial commissure droops. This leads to marionette lines and to the jowl becoming more pronounced.

When treating the jowl and marionette lines, sufficient knowledge of muscle and ligament anatomy and of changes in superficial and deep layers of fat is necessary (Fig. 5.23).

5.4.2 Injection and Methods

Both a needle and a cannula can be used to treat a marionette line. Treatment of marionette lines requires an injection into the medial portion of the wrinkle across multiple layers. Since drooping of the buccal fat pad is a significant cause in the formation of marionette lines, the injection must proceed with sufficient volume from deep to superficial layers. When injecting with a needle or cannula, the cross-hatching method is used to create sufficient volume (Figs. 5.24 and

5.25). Furthermore, a botulinum toxin injection into the DAO should accompany with filler injection treatment to improve the drooping of the lateral commissure, which often entails the formation of marionette lines. To reduce jowl, injection filler into prejowl sulcus can create smooth jaw line. However, in case of excessive fat volume of jowl or severe drooping, filler alone is not sufficient, so lifting procedure or fat removal besides filler injection can be helpful. Too much volume injection to Marionette line and prejowl sulcus can aggravate sagging appearance. Before injection, overall evaluation is necessary.

5.4.3 Side Effects

The facial a. and v., the inferior labial a. and v., and the mental a. and v. must be taken into consideration before proceeding with the injection. When finding the cannula insertion point, it is best to avoid the branching point of the facial a. (antegonial notch) and the mental foramen.

Fig. 5.24 Filler injection techniques for the Marionette line using cross-hatching injection by needle (**a**) and cannula (**b**) (Published with kind permission of © Kwan-Hyun Youn 2016. All rights reserved)

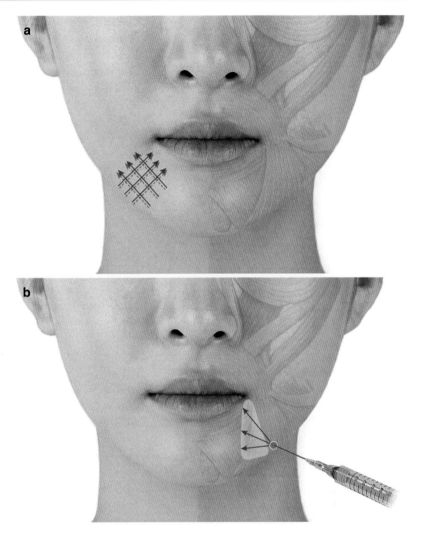

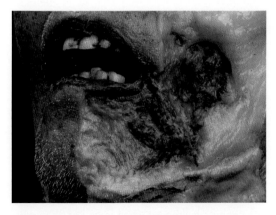

Fig. 5.25 The cadaveric filler injection for marionette line and hollow cheek (*dark green*) (Published with kind permission of © Hee-Jin KIm 2016. All rights reserved)

5.5 Anatomical Considerations of the Symptoms That May Accompany Filler Treatment

5.5.1 Vascular Compromise

Vascular compromise is one of the most severe side effects of filler injection, and a sound understanding of facial vascular anatomy can significantly reduce the risk of side effects. There are two reasons of vascular compromise, intravascular injection and external compression (Fig. 5.26).

First, filler products injected near vessel may cause the external pressure resulting in limited

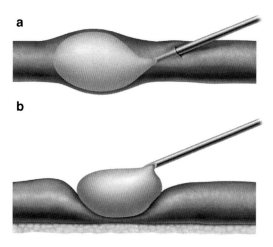

circulation of artery and can lead to localized or extended skin necrosis along the vessel flow depending on size of vessel compressed. External compression is more likely to occur when patients' skin is thick, firm and not movable, large amount of filler is injected into close to the skin, and excessive swelling after injection. The vulnerable vessels are supratrochlear a. on glabella, supraorbital a. on the forehead, lateral nasal a. on nose tip, dorsal nasal a. on the nose, and facial a. on NLF. So when injecting into the glabella, nose, and NLF, caution should be taken (Fig. 5.27). External compression of large vein can also cause skin necrosis via venous congestion, but it is not common. External compression by filler products is more common than intravascular injection.

Second, blockage of the vessel by intravascular injection of the filler products can occur and can lead to more serious problems. There are two intravascular injections, intravenous and intra-arterial injection.

First, vein-related side effects are usually due to venous congestion, and vein is more vulnerable to needle injury than artery due to thin and less elastic vessel wall. Unwanted injected filler particles may cause intravascular blockage of the vein, which generates much more severe venous congestion than external pressure on the vein. As time goes by without eliminating the etiology, venous congestion can affect capillary system and arterial circulation in order and finally cause the skin necrosis due to lack of circulation by arterial branches. The symptom by vein-related damage appears slowly; however, it is lighter than the artery-related damage. Nevertheless, in the case of intravascular injection into a vein, skin necrosis, pulmonary embolism, etc. may accompany. However, the exact mechanism by which pulmonary embolism occurs has not been confirmed.

On the other hand, in the case of arteries, intravascular injection rather than external pressure is the reason for embolism. Intravascular injection into the arteries can lead to skin necrosis by the embolism even within tens of minutes after the injection.

Injection into the arteries can lead to necrosis over a large area of skin, and the risk is greater to the end arteries. Skin necrosis can occur along the arterial pathway, and embolism can spread everywhere throughout the arterial branches, leading to severe side effects.

The most severe side effect of intravascular injection into arteries is loss of sight. Based on anatomic consideration, supraorbital a., supratrochlear a., and dorsal nasal a. from internal carotid a. and facial a. or angular a. from external carotid a. can continue to ophthalmic a. which nourishes the eye. Loss of sight can occur mainly due to intra-arterial injection of the filler. So high-risk regions for blindness are the glabella, the NLF, and the nose. The injected filler can traverse the arteries and can block the ophthalmic a., the central retinal a., and the post ciliary a. (Fig. 5.27). Furthermore, when injected with higher pressure, a large agglomeration of fillers injected may block the end artery.

Filler entry into arterial branches on the nose may also lead to blindness. Many cases of blindness after filler injection into the nose have been reported in Korea, and arterial injection has been reported to be the most common cause. When treating the tip of the nose or the dorsum of the nose, deep injection and aspiration can reduce the risk of intra-arterial injection. Use of a cannula is advised when injecting fillers into the nose; however, the risk of damaging arterial branches cannot be precluded.

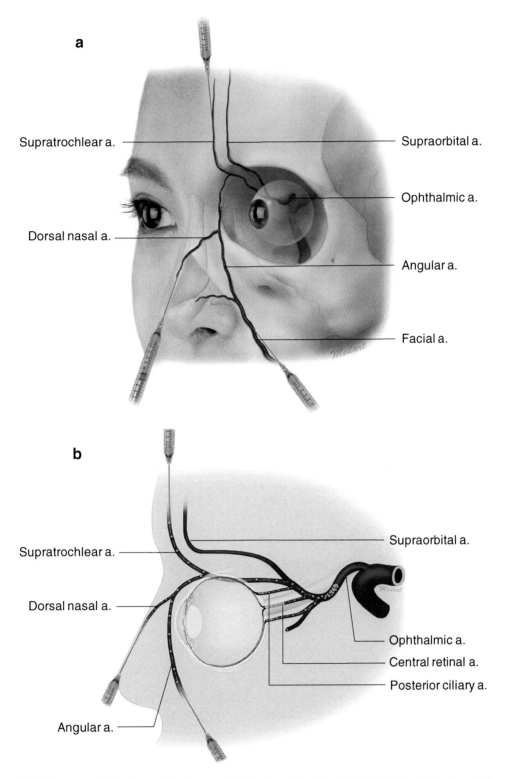

Fig. 5.27 The retrograde flow through the intra-arterial injection of the filler (**a**, **b**) (Published with kind permission of © Kwan-Hyun Youn 2016. All rights reserved)

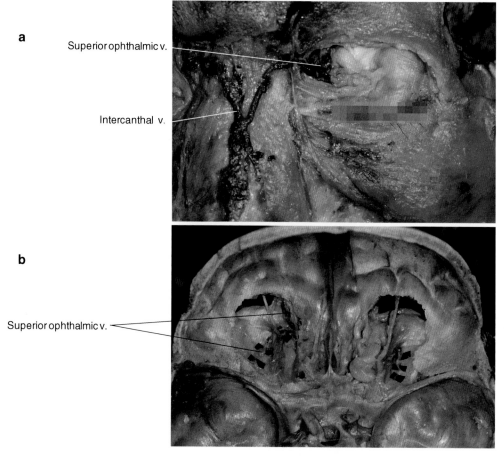

a

Superior ophthalmic v.

Intercanthal v.

b

Superior ophthalmic v.

Fig. 5.28 Vascular compromise by the puncture of the intercanthal vein using cannula (**a**) puncture of the intercanthal vein by cannula injection. (**b**) Location of the filler product at the cavernous sinus through the superior ophthalmic vein (Published with kind permission of © Hee-Jin Kim 2016. All rights reserved)

When injection starts with cannula from the tip of the nose, deep injection from tip to dorsum of the nose can be done; however, in some cases, cannula can be located into the subcutaneous layer at the radix rather than into the preferred layer just above the periosteum. In this case, vascular compromise by puncture of the venous structure such as the intercanthal vein may occur. Since the vessel walls of this vein are very thin and could easily be punctured by the cannula and needle, it is highly dangerous. There has been an actual case during a cadaver workshop when filler injections into the intercanthal vein lead to filler products partially traveling through the angular v. and the superior ophthalmic v. to the cavernous sinus (Fig. 5.28). Although it is hard to pinpoint the result of clinical problems, a possible consequence is a venous infection in the cavernous sinus, resulting in problems in arterial blood circulation through the venous congestion and the phlebitis. Therefore, when injecting fillers into the nose, aspiration prior to injection is vital even with cannula; furthermore, constant awareness of the tip of the needle or the cannula is pivotal.

5.5.2 Suggested Methods to Reduce Vascular Problems Related with Filler Injection

1. Small volume: Excessive amounts of filler should not be injected into one area. External pressure may increase causing damage to

blood vessels. Furthermore, intravascular injection of large amounts of filler may result in fatal consequences.

2. Slow injection: Any filler injection should proceed slowly. A slow injection can reduce the risk of damaging vessels by a sudden increase in pressure; furthermore, the chance of intravascular injection is also reduced.

3. Retrograde injection: Anterograde injection increases the chance of inadvertent intravascular injection.

4. Aspiration: Aspiration is the most effective method of verifying whether a needle or cannula is located within a vessel. Nonetheless, one cannot be absolutely certain that a needle or a cannula is not located within a blood vessel since no blood is withdrawn during aspiration. Furthermore, when using a filler of high viscoelasticity or when approaching a vessel of small diameter, aspiration may not be as effective.

5. Use of cannula: Using a cannula of relatively large diameter reduces the chances of intravascular injection; however, it does not ensure complete safety.

6. Size of the needle and cannula: Although there is controversy over this precaution, it is best to use a needle or cannula of sufficient size so that the pressure of injection is not high.

7. Anatomical knowledge: Above all, a thorough knowledge of the anatomy of the region being treated is necessary. Only a thorough knowledge of the location, depth, and pathways of arteries and veins can reduce the risk of side effects. Exact information of the vasculature in three-dimensional concept is mandatory to the filler injection.

Suggested Reading

Physical Anthropological Traits in Asians

1. Kim HJ, Kim KD, Choi JH, Hu KS, Oh HJ, Kang MK, Hwang YI. Differences in the metric dimensions of craniofacial structures with aging in Korean males and females. Korean J Phys Anthrop. 1998;11:197–212.

2. Youn KH, Kim YC, Hu KS, Song WC, Kim HJ, Koh KS. An art anatomical study of the facial profile of Korean. Korean J Phys Anthrop. 2002;15:251–62.

Muscles of the Face and Neck

3. Bae JH, Lee JH, Youn KH, Hur MS, Hu KS, Tansatit T, Kim HJ. Surgical consideration of the anatomic origin of the risorius in relation to facial planes. Aesthet Surg J. 2014;34(7):NP43–9.

4. Choi YJ, Kim JS, Gil YC, Phetudom T, Kim HJ, Tansatit T, Hu KS. Anatomic considerations regarding the location and boundary of the depressor anguli oris muscle with reference to botulinum toxin injection. Plast Reconstr Surg. 2014;134(5):917–21.

5. Hur MS, Hu KS, Cho JY, Kwak HH, Song WC, Koh KS, Lorente M, Kim HJ. Topography and location of the depressor anguli oris muscle with a reference to the mental foramen. Surg Radiol Anat. 2008;30(5):403–7.

6. Hur MS, Hu KS, Kwak HH, Lee KS, Kim HJ. Inferior bundle (fourth band) of the buccinators and the incisivus labii inferioris muscle. J Craniofac Surg. 2011;22(1):289–92.

7. Hur MS, Kim HJ, Choi BY, Hu KS, Kim HJ, Lee KS. Morphology of the mentalis muscle and its relationship with the orbicularis oris and incisivus labii inferioris muscles. J Craniofac Surg. 2013;24(2):602–4.

8. Kim HS, Pae C, Bae JH, Hu KS, Chang BM, Tansatit T, Kim HJ. An anatomical study of the risorius in Asians and its insertion at the modiolus. Surg Radiol Anat. 2014;37(2):147–51.

9. Yu SK, Lee MH, Kim HS, Park JT, Kim HJ, Kim HJ. Histomorphologic approach for the modiolus with reference to reconstructive and aesthetic surgery. J Craniofac Surg. 2013;24(4):1414–7.

Vessels of the Face and Neck

10. Koh KS, KIM HJ, Oh CS, Chung IH. Branching patterns and symmetry of the course of the facial artery in Koreans. Int J Oral Maxillofac Surg. 2003;32(4):414–8.

11. Kwak HH, Hu KS, Youn KH, Jin KH, Shim KS, Fontaine C, Kim HJ. Topographic relationship between the muscle bands of the zygomaticus major muscle and the facial artery. Surg Radiol Anat. 2006;28(5):477–80.

12. Lee JG, Yang HM, Choi YJ, Favero V, Kim YS, Hu KS, Kim HJ. Facial arterial depth and layered relationship with facial musculatures. Plast Reconstr Surg. 2015;135:437–44.

13. Lee SH, Gil YC, Choi YJ, Tansatit T, Kim HJ, Hu KS. Topographic anatomy of superior labial artery for

dermal filler injection. Plast Reconstr Surg. 2015;135: 445–50.

14. Lee SH, Lee M, Kim HJ. Anatomy-based image-processing analysis for the running pattern of the perioral artery for minimally invasive surgery. Br J Oral Maxillofac Surg. 2014;52(8):688–92.

15. Lee SH, Lee HJ, Kim YS, Kim HJ, Hu KS. What's difference between the inferior labial artery and horizontal labiomental artery? Surg Radiol Anat. 2015; 37(8):947–53.

16. Yang HM, Lee JG, Hu KS, Gil YC, Choi YJ, Lee HK, Kim HJ. New anatomical insights of the course and branching patterns of the facial artery: clinical implications regarding injectable treatments to the nasolabial fold and nasojugal groove. Plast Reconstr Surg. 2014;133(5):1077–82.

17. Yang HM, Lee YI, Lee JG, Choi YJ, Lee HJ, Lee SH, Hu KS, Kim HJ. Topography of superficial arteries on the face. J Phys Anthropol. 2013;26:131–40.

Peripheral Nerves of the Face and Neck

18. Hu KS, Yun HS, Hur MS, Kwon HJ, Abe S, Kim HJ. Branching patterns and intraosseous course of the mental nerve. J Oral Maxillofac Surg. 2007;65(11): 2288–94.

19. Won SY, Yang HM, Woo HS, Chang KY, Youn KH, Kim HJ, Hu KS. Neuroanastomosis and the innervation territory of the mental nerve. Clin Anat. 2014; 27(4):598–602.

20. Yang HM, Won SY, Lee JG, Han SH, Kim HJ, Hu KS. Sihler-stain study of buccal nerve distribution and its clinical implications. Oral Surg Oral Med Oral Pathol Oral Radiol. 2012;113(3):334–9.

Index

A

Alar band, wrinkle treatment, 75
Asian (Korean) skull and face
  aging process
    anatomy of, 48, 49
    facial appearance with, 50–51
    facial tissue, 49–50
  anthropological difference, 46
  brachycephalic shaped heads, 45
  symmetry, 47
  zygomatic bone, 47
Asians, nasolabial folds in, 129–131
Asymmetric smile, facial palsy
  injection points and methods, 74
  target muscle and anatomy, 72–74
Auriculotemporal nerve block (ATN block), 31, 32

B

BN block. *See* Buccal nerve block (BN block)
Botulinum toxin injection, 55
  effective *vs.* ineffective indications of, 56, 57
  facial contouring
    masseter hypertrophy, 84–87
    salivary gland hypertrophy, 88–89
    temporalis hypertrophy, 88–89
  rebalancing
    definition, 56
    elevators and depressors muscle groups, 58
    expression muscles, 56, 58
    mechanism of, 55, 56
    samurai eyebrow, 58
    side effect, 58
  Wrinkle treatment
    alar band, 75
    asymmetric smile, facial palsy, 72–74
    bunny lines, 69
    cobblestone chin, 80–81
    Crow's feet, 58–61
    drooping of, mouth corner, 75–80
    glabellar frown lines, 63–67
    gummy smile, excessive gingival display, 710
    horizontal forehead lines, 63–64
    infraorbital, 62–63
    nasolabial fold, 71–72
    platysmal band, 81–84
    plunged tip, of nose, 70–71
    purse string lip, 75–76
Breadth-height index, 46
Buccal artery, 35
Buccal nerve block (BN block), 29, 30
Bunny lines, wrinkle treatment, 69

C

Chin
  clinical anatomy, 160–161
  cobblestone, 80–81
  injection points and methods, 160, 162–164
  side effects, 162–165
Cobblestone chin, 80–81
Crow's feet
  botulinum toxin injection, 58–61
  face and neck, aesthetic terminology, 58–61

D

Depressor anguli oris muscle (DAO), 15, 16
Depressor labii inferioris muscle (DLI), 18
Depressor septi nasi muscle, 142–143
Dilator naris vestibularis muscle, 143
DLI. *See* Depressor labii inferioris muscle (DLI)
Dorsal nasal artery, 34
Dynamic wrinkles, 56

E

External nasal artery, 35

F

Face and neck
  aesthetic terminology
    aging facial creases and wrinkles, 2
    baggy lower eyelids and blepharochalasis, 2
    bunny and commissural lines, 3
    Crow's feet, 3
    facial creases, 2

© Springer Science+Business Media Singapore 2016
H.-J. Kim et al., *Clinical Anatomy of the Face for Filler and Botulinum Toxin Injection*,
DOI 10.1007/978-981-10-0240-3

Face and neck (*cont.*)
    festoon and gobbler neck, 3
    glabellar frown and transverse lines, 3
    horizontal forehead and neck lines, 3
    jowl and labiomandibular fold, 3
    marionette line, 3–4
    mentolabial creases and midcheek furrow, 4
    nasojugal groove and nasolabial fold, 4
    oral commissure, 3
    palpebromalar groove, 4
    periauricular lines, 4
    ptotic chin, 4
    skin folds, 2
    tear trough and temporal depression, 4
    vertical lip line, 4
  Asian (Korean) (*see* Asian (Korean) skull and face)
  blood vessels
    connections of vein, 42
    external carotid artery, 33
    facial artery, 35–38
    facial vein, 38–42
    internal carotid artery, 33, 35
    maxillary artery, 35, 36
    mental artery, 35
    ophthalmic artery, 34, 35
    retromandibular vein, 39, 42
    superficial temporal artery, 37, 39
    superficial temporal vein, 42
    veins with cutaneous nerves and artery, 38
  expressions and actions
    forehead region, 8, 11
    muscles, 5, 6, 9–10
    nose, 13–14
    orbital region, 11–12
    perioral muscles, 14–20
    platysmal muscles, 20
    SMAS (*see* Superficial musculoaponeurotic system (SMAS))
    temporal region, 7, 10, 11
  nerves
    ATN block, 31, 32
    BN block, 29, 30
    cutaneous sensory, 23
    GAN block, 31, 32
    IAN block, 31
    ION block, 28, 29
    lower face, 26–27
    midface, 25–26
    MN block, 29–30
    motor nerve, 26, 27
    sensory nerve, 26
    SON block, 28
    STN block, 28
    trunk of, 24
    upper face, 24–26
    ZTN block, 28, 29
  skin
    layers, 5–7
    thickness, 6, 7
  and skull surface landmarks, 42–45

Facial artery
  branches, 35–37
    angular artery, 37
    inferior alar branch, 36
    lateral nasal branch, 36–37
    of maxillary, 35, 36
    of ophthalmic, 34–35
    superior, inferior labial branch, 36
    typical distribution patterns, 37, 38
  nasolabial folds, in Asians, 129–131
Facial contouring, botulinum toxin injection
  masseter hypertrophy, 84–87
  salivary gland hypertrophy, 89–91
  temporalis hypertrophy, 88–89
Facial veins
  angular vein, 39, 41
  connections between, and angular vein, 42
  with cutaneous nerves and arteries, 38
  deep facial vein, 39
  external nasal vein, 39
  intercanthal vein, 39, 41
  labial vein, 39
  retromandibular vein, 39, 42
  superficial temporal vein, 42
Filler injection
  lower face for, 153–173
  midface for, 119–150
  upper face for, 93–117
Forehead and glabella
  clinical anatomy
    anatomical layers of, 96
    frontal eminence and concavity, 94–95
    hairline and eyebrows form, 94
    injection points and methods, 94–99
  side effects
    augmentation, 102
    dangerous injection plane, 102, 103
    glabellar wrinkles, 100
    skin necrosis, 100, 101
    use of cannula, 101
Frontoparietal index, 47
Frontozygomatic index, 47

G
GAN block. *See* Great auricular nerve block (GAN block)
Glabellar frown lines, 63–67
Great auricular nerve block (GAN block), 31, 32
Gummy smile, excessive gingival display, 71–72

H
Hollow cheek
  clinical anatomy, 135–137
  injection points and methods, 135, 138
Horizontal forehead lines, 63–66
Hypertrophy
  masseter, 84–87
  salivary gland, 89–91
  temporalis, 88–89

I

IAN block. *See* Inferior alveolar nerve block
    (IAN block)
Inferior alveolar nerve block (IAN block), 31
Infraorbital artery, 35
Infraorbital nerve block (ION block), 28–29
Infraorbital wrinkles, 62–63
Intercanthal vein (ICV)
    anatomy, 149
    distribution patterns and classification, 150
ION block. *See* Infraorbital nerve block
    (ION block)

L

Labial artery
    inferior, 159
    location of, 158
    superior, 158–159
Lacrimal artery, 34
LAO. *See* Levator anguli oris muscle (LAO)
Lateral orbital thickening, 23
Length-breadth index, 46
Length-height index, 46
Levator anguli oris muscle (LAO), 14, 16
Levator labii superioris alaeque nasi muscle (LLSAN),
    17, 18
Levator labii superioris muscle (LLS), 15–16, 18
Lips
    clinical anatomy, 154, 155
    injection points and methods, 154–157
    purse string, 75, 76
    side effects, 157–160
LLS. *See* Levator labii superioris muscle (LLS)
LLSAN. *See* Levator labii superioris alaeque nasi muscle
    (LLSAN)
Lower face, for filler injection, 153
    chin
        clinical anatomy, 160–161
        injection points and methods, 160, 162–164
        side effects, 162–165
    lip
        clinical anatomy, 154, 155
        injection points and methods, 154–157
        side effects, 157–160
    marionette line and jowl, 166
        clinical anatomy, 166–168
        injection and methods, 168, 169
        side effects, 168
    perioral wrinkles
        clinical anatomy, 165, 166
        injection points and methods, 166, 167
        side effects, 166, 167
    reduce vascular problems, 172–173
    vascular compromise
        cannula, 170, 172
        external compression, 169–170
        intravascular injection, 170
        by puncture, 172
        vein-related side effects, 170

M

Mandibular retaining ligament, 23
Marionette line and jowl, 166
    clinical anatomy, 166–168
    injection and methods, 168, 169
    side effects, 168
Masseter hypertrophy, 84–87
Masseteric cutaneous ligament, 23
McGregor's patch. *See* Zygomatic ligament
Mental artery, 35
Mentalis muscle, 18–19
Mental nerve block (MN block), 29–30
Midface, for filler injection, 119
    hollow cheek
        clinical anatomy, 135–137
        injection points and methods,
            135, 138
    nasojugal groove
        clinical anatomy, 124–126
        injection points and methods, 127–128
    nasolabial fold
        clinical anatomy, 128–131
        injection points and methods, 131–135
    nose
        clinical anatomy, 139–148
        injection points and methods, 148–150
    palpebromalar groove
        clinical anatomy, 128
        injection points and methods, 128
    subzygoma depression
        clinical anatomy, 138–139
        injection points and methods, 139, 140
    tear troughs
        clinical anatomy, 120–122
        injection points and methods, 123–124
MN block. *See* Mental nerve block (MN block)
Modiolus, 18, 20
    and converge muscles, 78
    muscles inserted into, 14, 16
    patterns and locations, 79
    tendinous structure of, 79
Motor nerve
    distribution of, 24
    lower face, 26, 27
    midface, 26
    upper face, 25, 26
Mouth corner, drooping of, 75, 77–80

N

Nasal index, 47
Nasalis muscle, 142
Nasojugal groove
    clinical anatomy, 124–126
    injection points and methods,
        127–128
Nasolabial fold
    clinical anatomy, 128–131
    injection points and methods, 131–135
    wrinkle treatment, 72–74

Nerves, face and neck
    ATN block, 31, 32
    BN block, 29, 30
    cutaneous sensory, 23
    GAN block, 31–32
    IAN block, 31
    ION block, 28–29
    lower face, 26–27
    midface, 25–26
    MN block, 29, 30
    motor nerve, 24
    sensory nerve, 24
    SON block, 28
    STN block, 28
    trunk of, 23, 24
    upper face, 24–26
    ZTN block, 28, 29
Nose
    clinical anatomy, 139–148
    injection points and methods, 148–150
    plunged tip of, 70–71

O
Ophthalmic artery, 34–35
Orbicularis retaining ligaments (ORL), 23, 120

P
Palpebromalar groove
    clinical anatomy, 128
    injection points and methods, 128
Paranasal muscles, 142
Perioral muscles
    dilators of, lips
        contracting muscle, of chin, 18–19
        labial commissure and midline, muscles inserted
            into, 15–18
        modiolus, muscles inserted into, 14–16
    intrinsic muscles, of lip and cheek, 14, 15
    layers, 19
Perioral wrinkles
    clinical anatomy, 165–166
    injection points and methods, 166, 167
    side effects, 166, 167
Platysma-auricular fascia (PAF), 23
Platysmal band, 81–84
Procerus muscle, 142

R
Risorius muscle, 15, 17

S
Salivary gland hypertrophy, 89–91
Sensory nerve
    cutaneous, 23
    distribution of, 24

    lower face, 26
    midface, 25
    upper face, 24
SMAS. See superficial musculoaponeurotic system
        (SMAS)
SON block. See Supraorbital nerve block (SON block)
Static wrinkles, 56
STN block. See Supratrochlear nerve block (STN block)
Suborbicularis oculi fat (SOOF), 124, 126
Subzygoma depression
    clinical anatomy, 138, 139
    injection points and methods, 139, 140
Sunken eye and pretarsal roll, for filler injection, 103
    clinical anatomy, 103–105
    injection points and methods, 105–109
    side effects, 109, 110
Superficial layer, lips, 19
Superficial musculoaponeurotic system (SMAS)
    layer and ligaments, of face, 21–22
        lateral orbital thickening, 23
        mandibular retaining, 23
        masseteric cutaneous, 23
        orbicularis retaining, 23
        platysma-auricular fascia, 23
        superior temporal septum, 21
        zygomatic, 23
        zygomatic cutaneous, 23–24
    layer, of skin, 5
Superior temporal septum, 21
Supraorbital artery, 34
Supraorbital nerve block (SON block), 28
Supratrochlear artery, 34
Supratrochlear nerve block (STN block), 28

T
Tear troughs
    clinical anatomy, 120–122
    injection points and methods, 123–124
Temple, for filler injection, 109–110
    clinical anatomy, 111–113
    injection points and methods, 113–116
    side effects, 116
Temporalis hypertrophy, 88–89
Transverse craniofacial index, 46–47
Transverse frontal index, 47

U
Upper face, for filler injection, 93
    forehead and glabella
        clinical anatomy, 94–96
        hairline and eyebrows form, 94
        injection points and methods, 94–99
        side effects, 100–103
    sunken eye and pretarsal roll, 103, 104
        clinical anatomy, 103–105
        injection points and methods, 105–109
        side effects, 109, 110

temple, 109–110
    clinical anatomy, 111–113
    injection points and methods, 113–116
    side effects, 116
Upper facial index, 46
Upper lip elevators, 18, 19

V

Vascular compromise
    cannula, 170, 172
    external compression, 169–170
    intravascular injection, 170
    by puncture, 172
    vein-related side effects, 170

W

Wrinkle treatment. *See also* Botulinum toxin injection
    alar band, 75
    asymmetric smile, facial palsy, 72–74
    bunny lines, 69
    cobblestone chin, 80–82
    Crow's feet, 58–62

drooping of, mouth corner, 75, 77–80
glabellar frown lines, 63–68
gummy smile, excessive gingival display,
        71, 72
horizontal forehead lines, 63, 64
infraorbital, 62–63
nasolabial fold, 71–74
platysmal band, 81–84
plunged tip, of nose, 70–71
purse string lip, 75–76

Z

ZMi. *See* Zygomaticus minor muscle (ZMi)
ZMj. *See* Zygomaticus major muscle (ZMj)
ZTN block. *See* Zygomaticotemporal nerve block
        (ZTN block)
Zygomatic artery, 35
Zygomatic bones, 47
Zygomatic cutaneous ligament, 22–23
Zygomatic ligament, 22
Zygomaticotemporal nerve block (ZTN block), 29
Zygomaticus major muscle (ZMj), 14, 16
Zygomaticus minor muscle (ZMi), 18

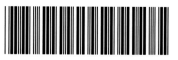